Caroline Carr

MENOPAUSE
The guide for
Real Women

IMPORTANT NOTE:

The information in this book is not intended as a substitute for medical advice. Neither the author nor White Ladder can accept any responsibility for any injuries, damages or losses suffered as a result of following the information herein.

This edition first published in Great Britain 2009 by
Crimson Publishing, a division of Crimson Business Ltd
Westminster House
Kew Road
Richmond
Surrey
TW9 2ND

A catalogue record for this book is available from the British Library.

ISBN 978 1 90541 057 6

Printed and bound by Ashford Colour Press Ltd, Gosport, Hampshire.

Acknowledgements

With love and respect to my own favourite Real Women: EG, GL and LEC.

Thank you so much to everyone who has contributed to this book. I am so grateful to those of you who shared your personal experiences, and to the professionals who gave me so much help and advice.

Contents

Introduction

I first heard the word 'menopause' when I was about 10, during an English lesson at school. We were taking it in turns to read aloud from a book. At one point our teacher stopped us and rose from her seat. She adjusted the long scarf that adorned her neck and looked at us intently for a few moments. Then she said: *'The menopause is a very special time, a very emotional time for a woman, you know.'* I had absolutely no idea what she was talking about.

Over the years I accumulated various bits of information from other girls, my mother, other people's mothers, and of course from magazines. As my life progressed, I gleaned more from health professionals, such as contraceptive advice, ante-natal advice, and post-natal advice. I only ever really found out as much as I needed to know at any given time. But it wasn't until I started the menopause process myself that I really took it seriously.

It is possible you are going through the menopause at the moment. Or you might be noticing changes within yourself and wonder if you are at the beginning of the whole process. This book will help you survive the menopause – whatever stage you are at.

If your own experience of the menopause is unlike anything mentioned here, then that's fine. Every woman is different – and that's what makes you unique.

How to use this book

This book explores each stage of the menopause. It tells you what is happening to your body and the initial changes you may notice. Then it looks at common issues that you might experience during the menopause, and other more serious possibilities that can occur.

Every issue covered is clearly explained and discussed, and includes a section called **What you can do to help yourself.** This gives practical tips on how to alleviate any discomforts and feel more accepting, positive and upbeat about this stage of your life.

The second section of the book deals with some of the treatments that are available. This will help you to weigh up the pros and cons of each treatment – from HRT to hypnotherapy. Then you can make informed decisions, and choose what is best for you.

There is also a section for your partner, to give them an insight into menopause and what you are going through. As this stage of your life will affect those closest to you, it's important that they are aware of what's happening to you and why.

Most of all, this is a book that will give you lots of practical tips and advice to use, and you will be able to read about other women's experiences.

Going through the menopause is not the end of the world. It's actually the start of a bright new phase of your life and having the right attitude to it will work wonders.

part one

Your approach

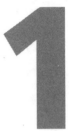

Preparing yourself for the menopause

Imagine you could choose when to have your menopause. I wonder what your choice would be. 'I'll have it now please, before my career really reaches its peak. I won't want to be bothered with it all then, so I'd like to get it out of the way.' Or how about, 'I'd prefer to wait for a few years until my children have grown up.' Or, 'It's not convenient right now. It looks like my husband is about to lose his job, and my mother is very frail. I'm going to have to spend more time looking after her. And my teenage son's behaviour is a worry, and my daughter's got her main exams coming up. I need to get all these things sorted out first, so I think I'll wait a while.' Or maybe, 'I've never wanted children and don't intend to have any, so what's the point of me having periods at all? I want my menopause now.' Or perhaps you'd say, 'I really do want to wait for about 25 years. I'm far too young to think about menopause yet.'

Wouldn't it be great if you could predict when it would occur, so that you could be prepared? But you can't.

For the majority of women, the menopause just seems to creep up, and often it isn't until the whole process is well under way that you realise that you are going through it.

For others, periods just stop without any warning, and then various other signs occur. Some women are thrown into the menopause as a result of treatment for an illness, or surgery. Some women – a very small percentage of the population – experience the menopause early, or even prematurely, possibly in their 30s, their 20s, or even younger.

In the same way, you cannot predict what changes you are likely to experience, or how severe they are likely to be, because this varies so much from one woman to another. You may just drift through the whole thing. On the other hand, you might have a rough time and feel absolutely terrible.

When does menopause occur?

In the UK the average age for a woman's final period is about 51 to 52. In some cases it may begin much sooner (possibly in your 30s) and end much later (you could be in your 60s), but it is usually somewhere between the ages of 45 and 55. The whole process can last for a few years.

The great thing is that there is plenty of help available, although the trick is knowing what would be right for you. There is support, whatever stage you may be at, and professional help. And there is so much that you can do to help yourself. So, whatever stage you are at, it is worth adopting a positive attitude, because menopause is not an illness, although it may feel as if it is sometimes. It's just a time of change.

The key thing is to understand what's happening to you, so that you can move forward with confidence, and feel in control.

Menopause: from the Greek *menos* (monthly), and *pausis* (ending).

This is the time when your periods stop. Your levels of the hormones oestrogen and progesterone fall, and your body stops producing eggs. Therefore you are no longer able to conceive naturally.

Perimenopause: This is the time leading up to the last period, and also the time after it – for about 12 months. You only really know that you are out of the perimenopause and into the next stage (postmenopause) when you have not had a period for 12 months.

Postmenopause: This is the time that starts after your last period. It is actually the whole of the rest of your life.

Climacteric: This term covers the whole lot. It refers to the whole transition and change.

THE MENOPAUSE IN OTHER CULTURES

Menopause happens. That's a fact. But in different cultures the experience of it varies. Some of this may be due to the diet and lifestyle differences, or to genes and environment. For example, in Japan, frozen shoulders often occur at menopause, which makes moving the upper body and arms tricky and painful. This is much more common than hot flushes, which are experienced far less in Japan and Asia than they are in the West.

> 66 In Malaysia we don't have the problems that you get at menopause. We hardly eat any dairy produce. You eat so much of it here. We do have cheese, but it's completely different, and it's not made from dairy. I drink soya milk and eat bean curd.
>
> Joo, 35 99

Studies have shown that many women may experience premature menopause because of malnutrition and poverty, for example in poor, rural areas of India. And in some areas of Latin America it is considered taboo to discuss menstruation and menopause, so girls and women aren't told about such things until they experience them. Therefore they worry that they are ill when changes in their bodies occur, or that there is a supernatural reason for them, and they may be treated with prayers and incantations or sent up a mountain to exorcise their demons.

In the West, menopause is seen as a natural time of transition and change for a woman, which can be managed and eased. It's an indication that you are approaching a new stage in your life. How you approach this transition is up to you.

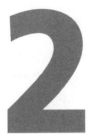

The importance of being positive

Years ago, not many women lived long enough to reach the menopause. If they did, they were invariably respected, honoured and considered wise. An attitude of respect towards older and post-menopausal women is still the case in some cultures and countries, but it may have been lost to a certain extent within the Western culture, where youth is often respected more highly than age.

Some women are very young when they go through the menopause, and this book is mindful of that. But the vast majority of women are in early middle age when changes start to occur.

> **"** Many older women want to look 40 for ever. There seems to be a fear of ageing, which I think is encouraged by the media. But being fit and healthy doesn't mean that you have to look young. I think that this desire to look and be young means that there's a tendency for some people to regard older generations as stupid, whereas a few generations ago they were considered to be the wise ones. Years ago, a post-menopausal woman was thought of as the Crone, that is, the Wise Woman, who people turned to for advice. But in many ways the Wise Woman has become disempowered now, because she hasn't kept up with technology. In this day and age, in order to be accepted in that position you have to keep up with technology and keep in touch.
> Anna, 63 **"**

With age comes confidence, even though this may plummet every now or then. Some of the changes brought about by menopause will have a lasting, profound effect. The physical changes may lead to those which are mental and emotional.

You may move through menopause with ease. You may experience some changes more than others, and adjust accordingly. Or you might feel as though you are being turned inside out, upside down, and thrown against a wall all at once.

But avoid viewing the menopause with dread. Yes, you may find some aspects uncomfortable, and you could feel emotional and perhaps question your role in life. You might lose confidence a little. You may not like the way you look, or the way you behave sometimes, or the way that you think and feel. You may potentially need some medical help. However, it is for you, remember:

The very best way that you can help yourself is to develop and sustain a positive attitude.

The way you think and feel about everything will make all the difference to your experience. Consider this: do you want to feel power*ful* or power*less*? If you are happy to feel powerless then I doubt you will have taken the time to read this book.

THE POSITIVES OF MENOPAUSE

Before exploring the possible changes you will encounter during menopause, this section lays out a few positive points about menopause. Whatever your age and wherever you are in the menopause process, sustaining a positive attitude is one thing that will see you through it. And you can help yourself by looking forward to the future, and finding the humour in situations. Holding the positive side of menopause in your mind can really help put things into perspective.

If you are a young woman experiencing a premature menopause, please avoid feeling affronted by this chapter. You will have specific concerns, and therefore some of the points made here may not seem relevant to you at this time. I hope that you will find chapter 7 on premature and early menopause useful, and respectful of your situation.

> **❝** Sometimes the menopause is a nuisance, but on the whole I quite like it. I feel like I'm being 'rounded off'. I just like the feeling of completing a whole area of my life. And then — well, who knows what I might do next?
> Benni, 50 **❞**

Your chance to make changes

While you are going through the menopause you get to go through your own personal transformation. It can be a time that presents an opportunity to change yourself – or perhaps an opportunity to make changes and adjustments in your life. You know that your body is changing, so this can be a great time to take stock and think things over. Many women have found that this is a good time to really consider what they want from life, and how they can give themselves the best possible chance of achieving it. But as your hormones run riot, you may feel overwhelmed, so it can be useful to have help with this.

Speaking to a life coach or mentor can help you get everything in perspective, as can talking to someone you trust who is objective and sensible, and who will listen to you and keep your best interests at heart.

It can also help to write things down, and you might like to do it like this:

PAST	PRESENT	FUTURE
Important life events	What is going on for you in your life right now?	How do you see your future?
Achievements – things that you are proud of and want to carry with you	How do you feel about it?	What do you want?
What you may want to leave behind	What are you thinking?	What would you really like to be doing?
	How are you helping yourself?	What do you need to do this?
	How might you not be helping yourself?	What of your own strengths and experiences can you draw on to help you?
	What would be the best thing for you right now?	

Periods

- However heavy or spasmodic your periods are, you can take heart from the fact that each one is one nearer to the last one you'll ever have. They are definitely on the way out, and are going to come to an end.

- The fact that you know that this is happening helps you to be clear that you are approaching another phase of your life. You can look forward to this as a new and exciting time, filled with all sorts of opportunities and possibilities.

> **❝** I was working too hard and felt as if I was on a hamster wheel, going round and round relentlessly. I was exhausted and I had no work/life balance at all. I felt really strongly that I just needed to stop and get myself into balance. So that's what I did. I decided to stop working full time. I knew that financially it could be tricky, but I thought 'I need time for myself now, and we'll just have to manage'. I reduced my hours at work by half, and I've never looked back. I feel much more relaxed now.
>
> And when you close one door another always opens. I started to write short stories for magazines and I've been very successful. It's great because I do this when I want to, and on my own terms. I get paid for doing something I love, and I have the control. **❞**
>
> Kathleen, 55

When your periods have stopped for good

No more periods

As you realise that your periods really *have* stopped for good, you may find yourself in a state of gentle euphoria as you start to appreciate all the benefits that this implies:

- You no longer have to spend any money on tampons or sanitary towels.

- You no longer have to be mindful of what day of the month it is in case your period starts.

- You no longer have to worry that you may stain the bed linen if you 'leak' during the night.

- You no longer have to carry sanitary paraphernalia around with you. Sanitary towels and tampons are no longer a part of your life. And you'll never need a 'special bin' again.

Contraception

Once you have well and truly been through the menopause, you don't need to use contraception any more. But do be clear about when it is safe to stop. See page 49 for more information.

Pampering

As you go through the menopause you have the perfect excuse for pampering yourself and trying out anything that enables you to feel better/well/fantastic. You can justify trying different therapies or spas or beauty treatments because you know you need to soothe yourself and feel good about yourself, and because you are worth it.

Rest

You have every right to have a rest now and then if you need it. You may have many things to do, but you will not do them effectively if you are exhausted. So if you want to take a rest – do so. Enjoy allowing yourself the time just to 'be'.

Excuses

You have the perfect excuse for almost everything. You can blame any emotion, or tiredness, or any forgetfulness, or irrational thought or behaviour on the fact that you are going through the menopause. And should you suddenly need to open a window, or leave the room, just tell others you are 'a little hot' or 'of that age', and they will probably leave you alone. The menopause provides a perfectly acceptable reason for all sorts of things. You might choose not to excuse yourself at all – but at least you have the option.

Some ailments clear up for good

Many women find that problems they had in the past improve or clear up completely during the menopause, so this could be something to really look forward to. For example, one woman said that she used to get spots on her face and back, but as she went through the menopause they started to clear up, and by the time her periods had stopped the spots had disappeared completely.

A woman who had been prone to awful migraines just before a period found that as her periods became less frequent, her migraines improved. By the time she had been through the menopause they went altogether.

Another woman said that she used to sweat a lot when she was younger and her clothes used to get very stained. When her periods stopped she found that the sweating stopped too.

Confidence and knowledge

Some women experience bouts of low self-esteem and a lack of confidence at some stages during the menopause process. If you recognise this in yourself, take strength from the fact that with the right attitude and mindset, your confidence will return. And when it does – wow! You will have more than you ever had before. You will feel comfortable and at ease with yourself – it really *is* possible.

❝ I don't feel compelled to do things I don't want to do any more, and if I get upset I tell myself that the feeling will go away. And eventually, it always does.
Lizzie, 54 **❞**

❝ I used to be embarrassed to be seen in a bathing suit at the beach or swimming pool. I felt everyone would think I was a great big clumsy lump. Since going through the menopause I don't give a damn. Why should I be bothered about what people think of my size and shape?
Renata, 65 **❞**

The wonderful thing about having confidence in yourself, and accepting who you are, is that you:

● Have the courage of your convictions.

● Are able to be assertive, and to say No when you want to.

● Feel able to tell others what they need to hear sometimes.

● Use your knowledge, skills and experience to help others when necessary.

● Feel compassion and express empathy, but not at the expense of your own well-being.

● Accept feedback graciously. You accept compliments without brushing them off. You also accept criticism without being offended, and you learn from it if it is well-founded.

- Feel gracious and easy with your place in the world. You accept that you have a perfect right to be there.

- Don't need to strive to impress others. You feel comfortable with what you know, and with what you have achieved.

- Are willing to seek help when necessary.

STEPS TOWARDS A POSITIVE APPROACH

Help yourself on the way to a positive outlook by making some clear decisions, and sticking to them:

Decide to take control

If you feel threatened by your reproductive cycle, you will be in conflict with it. If you view periods as something that *happens to* you, you will see your menopause in the same way. It too will *happen to* you. But you could choose to work with it, and see the whole process as a natural part of the woman you are and the person you have become. And once you've made that choice, you can decide how best to manage it, through seeking information and asking questions. This means that *you* take control. And how much better does that feel?

Decide to see this time as an opportunity

Draw on your experience of life (whatever your age) to inform and help others who have less understanding than you have.

Decide to turn everything to your advantage

Even if you are not happy with the way things are, you can come out on top if you want to. And the method is simple – always look for the benefits, because there will be some. For example, if you feel terrible – perhaps you have anxiety attacks – you *can* do something about it. As you find ways of coping, you ultimately develop yourself. It may not seem that way at the time, but just accept that it is so. You will reap the benefits later.

Decide not to give yourself a hard time
Instead of beating yourself up, accept things as they are – and move on.

Decide not to let others put upon you
Tell them how it makes you feel when they do, and then tell them what you would like to happen. You may be pleasantly surprised by their reaction.

Decide to ask for help if you need it
Know what you want help with and choose the best person to ask, and then – ask them.

Decide to keep a sense of perspective
Step back from the detail occasionally and slow down so that you get a bigger view. If you feel irritated or overwhelmed, just stop for a moment. Acknowledge that this is how you think and feel *right now*, and that it's OK to do so. You may think and feel differently later on. Distract yourself by focusing for a while on something that pleases you. Give your time, attention and energy to that. You could go for a walk, talk to a friend, read or write a story, do some exercise, or just make a cup of tea. Then you can look at the situation afresh.

Decide to look your best
This will help you to feel confident. Whatever your style, keep your nails, shoes and hair in good order. It makes such a difference. Your hair texture may change, and if your once flowing, curly chestnut locks now resemble a mouse-coloured pan scourer, it may be an idea to do something about it. And avoid dressing

frumpily. It's so easy to let yourself go when you feel bad, but making a bit of effort can actually have an effect on how you feel inside.

Decide to walk tall

Check your posture and avoid slouching. Hold yourself upright, but not too tense. If you sit and stand tall and with ease, you will look good and feel more graceful anyway. You may have been carrying lots of tension in your neck and shoulders, so it's a good idea to release them from time to time – just let your shoulders drop. If you learnt to slouch or hunch your shoulders when you were younger because you were tall, or because you had a large bust, now is the time to change, and acknowledge your rightful place in the world.

Decide to feel pleased with yourself

Acknowledge the things that you've achieved and done well in your life, and be proud of them. Avoid worrying if you find this tricky, because it's quite common to struggle with this, particularly if you feel low and your confidence has taken a knock. So give yourself time. Something will come to you. And when it does, you'll start to notice even more things that you can add. There are lots of reasons why you should feel pleased with yourself.

Decide to smile and to keep upbeat

A scowling, bad-tempered face is far less attractive than a smiling, accepting one.

Decide to be informed

So that you can choose how best to deal with the changes as they occur.

All these things can give you such a boost, yet they are relatively simple to do.

Say what you mean

When asked how you feel, how often do you answer 'I'm fine!' yet really mean that you're **F**razzled, **I**nsecure, **N**eurotic and **E**xasperated?

If this resonates with you, perhaps now is the time to ask yourself why. Might it be because you don't want to offend others? Or perhaps you feel unable to say how you really feel. The thing is, you may not be helping yourself by bottling things up. So find ways of saying what you need to say in a way that is respectful of everyone involved. For example, you might like to try the step-by-step approach on page 20, because this can be a great way of getting your point across – and, sometimes, of getting what you want!

❝My biggest plea is for women to keep a balance and see the menopause as a positive time to look forward. There's no reason why you can't continue to live a very full and happy life, but if you are having problems, then there are treatments out there that can help you.

Tim Hillard, consultant gynaecologist, chairman of the British Menopause Society **❞**

Julie

Julie has a very no-nonsense, down-to-earth approach to menopause. She's now 68 and tells her story.

"I can't really say that it bothered me at all. I had a hysterectomy when I was about 52 because I had a prolapsed womb after I'd had four children. I think my ovaries were left in place. I wasn't offered any HRT or anything, and having the hysterectomy was the best thing I ever did.

"As far as symptoms go, I had no hot flushes during the day – ever. But at night, I'd wake and the bed would be soaking wet, and I would be too. My husband would say I was terrible at menopause, and that he couldn't say anything to me because I was very tetchy. But I don't think I was.

"I've always accepted that period pain is just one of the things you have to go through, and there's no point in worrying about it. My attitude is the same with the menopause. You just have to go through it because it's what happens, so it's best just to get on with it. It isn't always pleasant, but just keep going and go through it. I'm way past that time now. Periods are a distant memory, which is marvellous. But I'm very active and do lots of things that I love. I think if you've got things to look forward to, you haven't the time to dwell on how you feel."

Annette

Annette *is a 55-year-old mother of four. She started the menopause at the age of 50 and found the process had a profound effect on the way she thinks and feels, as she's gained more confidence along the way.*

"My periods changed about five years ago. They'd be far less frequent, the flow was lighter, and sometimes there was a change in colour – more brown than red. I haven't had a period for about 18 months now.

"I had hot flushes - I'd notice a sort of tingling on my face and just more warmth about me. When you walk about you probably don't notice that you're going hot and cold so much, because the air moves past your face. But they weren't bad, and I never needed to take anything. I still have hot flushes a bit now, but not much.

"I feel generally achey in the morning, and I wake up in the night far more than I used to. I don't sleep in the same bed as my husband any more, because he's such a light sleeper.

"I'm also aware that my memory is getting a lot worse. So now I keep my mobile phone by my bed, and if I wake up in the night and remember something, I immediately put a message on the calendar on my phone, then I can go back to sleep. I sometimes do my pelvic floor exercises if I wake up in the night, and that sends me to sleep. I suppose I'm concentrating - like counting sheep.

"Now, I feel less at the mercy of everyone's emotions. I feel aware, and in control, and can just sit and listen and observe. Now I think: 'I don't have to be a certain person to this person, or in this situation. What goes on around me doesn't have to affect me. I don't have to change myself to adapt to them.'

"With the menopause, some women do have a rough time and it's appropriate to see your doctor if you're concerned. But the menopause is a natural thing, and it's going to happen, so don't bury your head in the sand. Find out about it yourself, and then you'll know what you might expect."

part two

What happens?

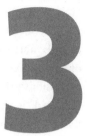

Your menstrual cycle

This chapter tells you how you arrive at your menopause. It's the technical bit. You may know a lot of this already – or you may not. It's designed to refresh your memory and put the next few chapters in context. You may be surprised how much you don't know about what goes on in your body. It is pretty amazing.

THE BASICS

When you were born you had about a million potential little 'eggs' in your ovaries already. You might have known that, but did you know that you had even more when you were a 12-week-old foetus in the womb? You had about two million potential eggs then. The vast majority of these cells decrease steadily throughout your life, so that when you approach menopause the number left is actually very small.

Most women will have approximately 12 menstrual cycles per year between the ages of about 14 and 50. In each cycle, a number of cells start to develop into eggs and, in theory, only the best one wins. The rest shrivel and fade away. Then, as you know, if each month the winning egg doesn't meet a sperm and become fertilised, it will leave your body along with blood and womb tissue – and you have a 'period'.

Eventually egg production stops altogether. And when that happens, you have the menopause – part of a perfectly natural sequence of events.

The next sections deal with glands and hormones. You may be very familiar with these, and if so, you will be aware of the huge part they play not only at puberty and at your menopause, but throughout your entire life. At puberty, it's as if everything is switched on. Some of your glands and hormones start to act slightly differently, so that you begin to develop into a young woman. That's when the whole process that will end in menopause is put in place.

Of course, it's not *just* about hormones and glands. Bodies are complicated mechanisms, with all sorts of systems at work. Everything interacts and works together for the good of the whole, so that when something in one 'system' or area is affected in some way, it is bound to impact on everything else.

GLANDS AND HORMONES

Everyone, regardless of sex or age, has hormones and glands. Both are essential and are absolutely fundamental to your health and well-being. Amongst other things, they work to help your body to achieve a level of balance and equilibrium. Therefore, glands and hormones are completely connected to every aspect of your health at all stages of your life.

Glands

Different glands do different jobs, depending on what type they are. Basically, they are responsible for producing and releasing various essential substances into your body.

There are two main types:

Exocrine glands
These release what they make into ducts or cavities inside the body, and then in some cases to its outer surface. Some of these glands are found near the skin, the tongue, the genitals, the eyes, the stomach and the throat. Some of the substances they produce are sweat and mucus.

Endocrine glands
These make hormones, which they release straight into the bloodstream. Some endocrine glands multi-task, because they do other things too. And some of them release what they make into ducts as well. For example, the pancreas produces digestive enzymes which it secretes into ducts to help with digestion, as well as making hormones and releasing them directly into the bloodstream.

Because endocrine glands produce hormones, they are directly relevant to the menopause. So here's some information about the main ones:

The pituitary gland
This is about the size of a pea and is situated at the base of your brain. It is called the 'master gland' because it controls many of

the other endocrine glands. It also produces hormones, which have a range of functions.

The pineal gland

Also in your brain, this gland produces melatonin, a hormone which is thought to be affected by the daily pattern of light and darkness. It is therefore thought to have an effect on waking and sleeping patterns and on how changes in the season may affect you.

The thyroid gland

This gland is in your neck and is one of the largest endocrine glands. The hormones it produces affect growth and the rate of metabolism, including the use of energy. The four parathyroid glands behind it produce a hormone that regulates blood-calcium levels.

The thymus

The thymus gland is in your chest. The hormones it produces stimulate the production of certain infection-fighting cells. It works hard from babyhood until puberty when it becomes very large. Then it steadily decreases in size, until in old age it almost disappears.

The adrenal glands

Positioned on each kidney, the adrenal glands produce several hormones that influence the way your body responds to stress. They also have an effect on metabolism.

The pancreas

The hormones that the pancreas produces control glucose levels in your blood.

The ovaries

The ovaries produce the hormones progesterone and oestrogen, which are also referred to as the female sex hormones because they are essential to sexual development and fertility.

The equivalent of these in males are the testes, which produce the hormone testosterone, referred to as the male sex hormone because it too is essential to sexual development and fertility. The ovaries also produce a small quantity of testosterone in females.

The hypothalamus

The hypothalamus is the area of your brain that appears to control the whole lot, starting with the pituitary gland. It's about the size of an almond. The hypothalamus is thought to control a large number of automatic bodily functions, including your body's biological clock, body temperature, hunger and food intake, thirst, the balance of water and salt in your body, tiredness, blood flow, and the way you respond to various emotions such as fear, stress and anger. It produces some hormones, too. It is situated in the middle of the base of your brain, where the nervous and hormonal body systems interact. More on the hypothalamus later.

The main thing to realise about glands is that they are very important, they have several essential functions within the body, and that some (the endocrine glands) produce hormones.

Hormones

You may know a great deal about hormones but if you don't, it's worth spending a few minutes reading this section because there may be more to hormones than you think.

❝ I'm so emotional. I cry at the drop of a hat. I suppose it's my hormones.
Marie, 54 **❞**

- Hormones basically run your life. There are many different ones and they all have specific jobs to do.

- They are chemicals which are made in different places in your body, and some hormones are made in several different places – in varying amounts. From there they go straight into your bloodstream.

- Think of them as the body's chemical messengers. Too much or too little of each can cause an imbalance in the body so that you may notice a range of physical symptoms and changes, or you may feel unwell.

- Their overall job is to keep you healthy and in balance. So if the level of one hormone decreases, others will rally round to help (but sometimes they may overdo it a bit).

- There's lots of interplay and interaction between different hormones, such as sex hormones, thyroid hormones and adrenal hormones. So the aim is to keep everything working well. It's a bit like fine-tuning an orchestra.

- A hormone targets only the cells which have specific receptors for that particular hormone. You have receptors in all areas of your body – for example, in your bones, in your brain, your gut, your breasts and womb.

Some of the reasons why hormones are so important are that they have an effect on your:

- Immune system, and on how it works.

- Metabolism and energy levels.

- Growth and development, from cells to baby to child to teen to adult.

- Mood, and therefore how you think and feel about things. It follows that they must therefore have an effect on how you behave.

- Libido and how sexy you feel.

- Skin, hair, gums, how much you sweat, how much mucus you produce, how watery your eyes get, and so on.

- Muscles, how they work, and how cells die off – which is a continuous process.

They contribute towards balance and equilibrium in your life, by preparing you to:

- Deal with an emergency or a trauma. This is when the stress response (or fight/flight mechanism) kicks in so that you will be able to cope.

- Deal with any new challenge or disruption, such as a sudden change in temperature or an infection.

- Cope with changes in life such as puberty and menopause.

They control the entire reproductive cycle, contributing to:

- Sperm and egg production

- Fertilisation

- Nourishment of the embryo

- Development of the foetus

- The birth

- Breastfeeding

Hormones affect every part of your life, whether you are male, female, child or adult. They help to regulate everything in your body, and to keep you in mental, physical and emotional balance – although there are times when this may not appear to be the case, for example when certain hormones seem to be surging relentlessly, such as during puberty and the menopause, or when things are not working as efficiently as they might be.

Hormones and glands working together

To get an overall idea of how the hormones and the glands all work together, you might like to think of your body as a large company. At the top is the hypothalamus, who oversees everything and delegates:

- Imagine the hypothalamus is the company director. She sits there all the time, keeping an eye on things.

- When she is disturbed, she contacts (by sending out hormones) her personal assistant (the pituitary gland), and tells her to deal with the situation.

- The pituitary gland jumps to attention and sends out hormones, each of which has a particular job to do. Some will start to deal with the situation directly. Others will send messages to different departments (various endocrine glands, and other sites in the body), telling them to manufacture their hormones immediately.

- As soon as the hormones are produced, they get to work straight away, doing whatever job they are assigned to do.

- This process is carefully monitored by a quality control system, so that each hormone is produced at the correct level, depending on which job it is going to do.

Quality control is a feedback process which works like this:

Negative feedback loop

When enough of the required hormones have been produced, the message is sent to the company director that it is time to stop. And so the balance is returned, and the job is done.

Positive feedback loop

If more of a particular hormone is needed, the message is sent to the company director to that effect. For example, the level of one hormone might be too low, so you need some more. Similarly, if you are coping with an emergency situation, you'll need specific hormones at higher levels for a time to help you to get through. And then when it's all over, the negative feedback loop should kick in and send back the message that it's time to stop.

But sometimes, if quality control isn't working efficiently, and the hormone production isn't regulated, some hormones may be produced in larger quantities than are needed. The whole point of the feedback loop is to help the body to maintain a balance.

Puberty

The first time you were probably aware of hormonal activity was at puberty, when changes started happening to your body. Your periods started and your shape began to change, along with the development of underarm and pubic hair. The main hormone responsible for this was oestrogen.

Suddenly, you had hormones in your body in amounts that you were not used to, and you'd never experienced anything quite like it before. You weren't used to the barrage of chemical information that was rushing around inside you. So as your body worked to adjust to the fluctuating hormone levels, your mood probably fluctuated too. You may have felt really high sometimes, and extremely low at others – but had no idea why.

Testosterone is also produced in small amounts by the adrenal glands, and also the ovaries, which is why females have some testosterone in their bodies too. It aids health and well-being.

So huge hormonal changes occur at puberty which affect not only physicality but also moods and emotions. This is bound to be the case, because hormones are linked to *everything* – the physical, mental and emotional aspects of a person.

HOW THE MENSTRUAL CYCLE WORKS

Your menstrual cycle is integral to your entire life. It is part of you each day, every day for all the time between puberty and the menopause.

Understanding this will help you to understand your menopause. Many women tend to think of the menstrual cycle in terms of the days leading up to, and during, a period only.

But it is a continuous process, except when there is a break during pregnancy or if your cycle is disturbed by other things, such as an illness or emotional upset. And of course, there are all sorts of differences and complications from woman to woman. For example you may have extremely heavy periods, or they may be spasmodic. Every woman is unique, and so the following couple of sections are a basic and very general explanation of what happens during your menstrual cycle:

- It starts with a period.

- Then a new egg develops in an ovary.

- After about 14 days the egg leaves the ovary and wanders off along a fallopian tube towards the womb.

- When it gets to the womb it disintegrates and leaves the body with blood and some of the lining of the womb. That's the end of your period, unless the egg was fertilised along the way.

- And then it all starts again.

This is a continuous, daily process from the moment your body starts preparing for your very first period until you have your last one at the menopause.

Therefore, the way you think, feel and behave is inextricably linked with your menstrual cycle. It's not just a matter of how you feel around the time of your period – it's all the time.

As different quantities of hormones are produced at different times in your cycle, there are bound to be various changes – physically, emotionally and mentally, depending on whereabouts in your cycle you are. When one hormone level rises, another falls, while others remain relatively consistent. The rise and fall can be dramatic because the hormones have different jobs to do.

Hormones in the menstrual cycle
There are four main hormones to consider in the menstrual cycle:

- Oestrogen.

- Progesterone.

- Follicle stimulating hormone (FSH).

- Luteinising hormone (LH).

They are known collectively as the female sex hormones.

Oestrogen

Both women and men produce the steroid substance oestrogen in their bodies, but women produce it in vastly larger quantities, especially from puberty onwards. There are several types, which is why they are often referred to as oestrogens, but usually they are collectively called oestrogen.

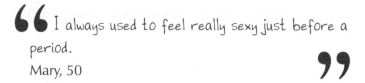 I always used to feel really sexy just before a period.
Mary, 50

Oestrogen is produced in small quantities in several different places in the body, but in females most of it is produced by the ovaries, and there are oestrogen receptors all over the female body, including the brain, breasts, heart, blood vessels, uterus, vagina, bladder, liver, bones, skin, and the digestive system.

It is one of the main female sex hormones, involved in all matters connected with menstruation, sex, reproduction and the menopause. It also is responsible for the development of secondary female characteristics, such as growing breasts, larger hips possibly, and pubic and underarm hair. And then it has an effect on a whole range of other things, such as skin and hair.

Apart from all the 'girlie' things that oestrogen does, it has masses of other functions, as it affects the heart, the bones, the blood, the immune system, the brain (including how efficiently your brain works, how you co-ordinate your movements, and how you perceive pain).

So oestrogen is a very important hormone for women, and how an individual responds to it varies. It's not until something happens, such as the levels change, or it's not working as efficiently as it might be, that you realise just how important it is and how much it influences what you do.

Progesterone

Both men and women produce the steroid substance progesterone – but men produce very little. In fact women produce very little, except when they are of an age when their reproductive system is working. It is one of the main female sex hormones, produced in a range of places, but particularly in the ovaries and the womb.

Among other things, it affects the nervous system, muscles, blood, bones, thyroid function, and the brain. But its main jobs are to regulate the effects of oestrogen and stop it getting out of control, and to prepare the lining of the womb for pregnancy.

For example, oestrogen makes the lining of the womb grow, and progesterone gets it ready for pregnancy. Then, as the level of progesterone falls, the lining of the womb comes away and you get rid of it (via a period). That is, if there is no fertilised egg. However, if there *is* a fertilised egg in the womb, progesterone will ensure that it is supported and helped along its way.

Follicle Stimulating Hormone (FSH)

Both men and women produce FSH. It is made in the brain by the pituitary gland. In males it stimulates the production of sperm, and in females its job is to make the follicles (eggs in their sacs) grow.

Luteinising Hormone (LH)

Both men and women produce LH. It is also produced by

the pituitary gland. In males it stimulates the production of testosterone, and in females it helps the follicles (eggs in their sacs) to pop out of the ovaries.

Testosterone

Both men and women produce the steroid substance testosterone. As it's the main male sex hormone, males produce much more – and mainly in their testes, whereas it's made mainly in the ovaries in females. It is important for general well-being, affecting bones, brain, muscles, mental and physical energy levels, and sex drive. It can also affect body odour.

What happens during the menstrual cycle

On day one, which is the start of the menstrual cycle, **the oestrogen and progesterone levels *start off low*,** and the lining of the womb sheds, so you have a period.

At the same time, **the pituitary gland starts releasing FSH *to a high level*.** This triggers follicles (eggs in their sacs) to start maturing in your ovaries.

As the follicles grow, they release increasing amounts of **oestrogen.** This *builds up sharply* as the egg is growing, as its main job is to make the lining of the womb grow and thicken enough to comfortably house a fertilised egg.

The big climax comes at around day 14, during a mass of hormonal activity. **Once the oestrogen reaches a certain level, it triggers the pituitary gland to release a *surge of LH*,** which causes the most mature follicle to pop its egg into the fallopian tube. This is ovulation – the result of 14 days of hard hormonal work.

As soon as that egg is released **LH rapidly drops to a *low level*** because it has finished its job for that month, and the **oestrogen** level *drops sharply*, although it is still there at a lower level supporting everything.

At the same time, **FSH *decreases fairly gradually*** to a low level for a while.

Meanwhile, as soon as the egg is released, the empty follicle produces **progesterone** as well as continuing to produce a certain level of **oestrogen**. The **progesterone level shoots *right up*** to support the egg in case it has been fertilised. Its main job is to prepare the lining of the womb for this and to modify the level of oestrogen, because otherwise the womb lining would just carry on growing.

At the same time, the level of **FSH begins its *gradual rise*** ready to start the follicles maturing again.

If the egg is not fertilised the follicle breaks down and **stops** producing hormones. By now the level of **progesterone *falls dramatically* to join the already low level of oestrogen.** And so the womb sheds its lining again and you have another period.

If you were not already familiar with the details of all this hormonal activity during the menstrual cycle, you might find looking at a graph is useful. There are some great ones on the internet, which can easily be found through the search engines.

The reason a graph can be helpful is that it gives a good indication of how really steeply the hormone levels rise and fall. It can be like looking at a high, steep mountain range. In any case, just bear these words in mind to remind you: *peaks and troughs, rise and fall dramatically, rise and fall gradually, shoots up steeply, plunges sharply, maintains a steady level.* Because this is what hormones do.

> ❝ By the third day, I felt like I'd been 'cleansed' – reborn. It was like a fresh start each month.
> Ellen, 49 ❞

As an adult you might cope with dramatic changes in hormone levels relatively easily because it's a familiar experience to you. If you are used to this experience, you probably accept it. This doesn't necessarily mean that you enjoy it, but you can deal with it. Similarly, when the weather changes completely from one day to the next, you may just notice and think: "Oh it's raining today" or 'It's a sunny day'. It may not bother you too much.

> ❝ A glass of gin and tonic used to sort me out each time.
> Jennie, 63 ❞

On the other hand, you might react in a more extreme way, and think 'Oh my God it's raining – it's the end of the world.' In the same way, if your hormone levels are fluctuating dramatically, or if your body is not producing enough of an individual hormone, or too much of another, you can feel terrible – and often very low. So you may have terrible mood swings, and behave in a way that is completely out of character when you are pre-menstrual. For example, there have been cases of women shoplifting, and there was an extreme example of one woman who attempted suicide each month at a particular time in her menstrual cycle.

A woman's life is her cycle.

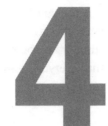

The early stages of the menopause

As you get older the quality and quantity of your eggs begins to diminish. In other words, they are not as good and there are not as many as there were. It's as if your ovaries just can't be bothered to produce anything. So they make less oestrogen and progesterone, and then your periods stop. They may grind to a halt gradually over time, or they may stop suddenly. Either way, this happens naturally as part of the natural process of reaching the end of your reproductive life.

But for some women, menopause occurs because of some medical treatments and operations – for example, if your ovaries are removed, or if you have had chemotherapy or radiotherapy. Some medical conditions can also trigger menopause, and so can some illnesses and infections. And, you may have an early, or a premature, menopause. (There's more about this in chapter 7.)

It is thought that the falling levels of oestrogen cause the most havoc, because oestrogen has so many other functions apart from stimulating the release of eggs. But it's important to remember that everything works together – hormones interlink and help each other out.

The tiniest changes in one part of your body can have an effect physically, mentally and emotionally on all the rest – even though you may not be aware of it.

HOW DO YOU KNOW YOU ARE MENOPAUSAL?

There's no simple answer to this question. Unless it all happens very suddenly, you might be in the lead-up to it (the perimenopause) for years without realising it. And although age is an indicator, it can't be completely accurate because every woman is so different. Currently in the UK the average age for the final period is about 51 or 52. But you could have been building up to this for years. On the other hand, you may still be having regular periods when you're 56, and not be aware of any symptoms at all.

66 I seem to view things in a different light, and I'm noticing odd things. I often feel unusually emotional, such as when I'm watching the news. Things really get to me now, and I sometimes cry.
Rebecca, 43 99

You might just get used to the way that you feel from one day to the next, and not give it much thought. Perhaps you notice subtle changes, such as the odd ache here and there, a lighter period every now and then, or feeling fed up. Maybe you tell yourself you're just getting a bit older and then forget about it. Or you might be aware of a variety of changes, some of which are unpleasant and inconvenient.

 ❝ I still have regular periods, but they're much lighter than they used to be. I don't think I get hot flushes as such, but now I blush when I start talking or give a presentation, and that makes me hot and sticky. It's ridiculous, because I've done presentations all my life, and now suddenly, I can feel the colour coming up and it's so embarrassing. I haven't blushed since I was about 14. ❞

Claire, 54

Talking to someone who knows about the menopause will help. Your doctor or nurse is a good person to start with, and depending on your age and the changes you notice, he or she will be able to advise you and to suggest ways forward. They might decide to do a test which will determine whether or not you are in the menopausal process – but this may not be necessary. And there are some home kit tests that you can do for yourself, but these are not always accurate.

Menopause clinics

Some areas have menopause clinics, or something similar, which are run by specialists. These are great, because you can find out all you need to know from people who really know about it. They are run differently in different areas, and sometimes you can just go along for a chat, but others need a referral from a GP or a practice nurse. The great thing is that whereas a GP may only have about five minutes to talk to you, the chances are that you will get more time at a menopause clinic – maybe 15 minutes or a bit longer. Ask your GP or practice nurse for your nearest clinic.

❝ Most women just want information and a chat, and to go through what's happening to their bodies. They want to know what's likely to happen in the future and how they can help themselves. And they want to know what treatments are available. These can include complementary therapies through to HRT, and though I can't recommend complementary therapies, I can tell them what some women have found useful. Most women want to know how long the whole process will last — and unfortunately there's no answer to that. Lots of women come early on, because they want to have the information and knowledge base, but some only come when they experience problems.

The majority of women want a holistic approach. They want to feel that someone is listening to them and taking them seriously. And they want to get their questions answered. Just going to the doctors' surgery and being written out a prescription is not helpful. A lot of things come to a head at menopause. Often women have coped with all sorts of things for years, and then they get to menopause and sometimes specific counselling is required.

Amanda Hillard, clinical nurse specialist who runs a menopause clinic **❞**

Contraception

One of the things that you might want more information about is contraception, because as you approach, experience and move past the menopause, this can be utterly confusing. The guidelines about this are:

- If you are over the age of 50 and your periods have stopped for a year, you should continue to use contraception for another year after that.

- If you are under the age of 50 and your periods have stopped for a year, you should continue to use contraception for a further two years.

This sounds simple, but of course you may not be able to remember when your last period was. With everything else that goes on during the menopause process, the date of your last period may have faded into the background. Hormone Replacement Therapy (HRT) is not contraception, and if you are taking this you will still need to use something. But take advice on what will be the best method for you. Also, if you are having irregular periods you still need to use contraception.

COMMON INDICATORS OF THE MENOPAUSE

Gradual changes and decreases in hormone levels will bring about all sorts of subtle changes, which you may hardly notice as you slowly adjust over time. But you might find yourself thrown into physical, emotional and mental disarray as your hormones appear to have a wild party – at your expense.

The changes you are likely to notice will vary as you go through menopause, so just be aware of this. The other thing to be aware of is that you may not realise that your menopause is beginning to happen. Very often, you might look back after a few years and think: 'So that's what all that was about.'

You might find that:

- You feel more emotional sometimes, or even have real mood swings.

- You get more tired than you used to – in fact you might feel exhausted and drained sometimes, and feel that you have lost your spark and zest for life.

- You notice that your periods have changed, and maybe you've missed a few.

- You have the odd ache and pain that you've never had before.

- You have bladder problems or infections, and maybe you sometimes worry that you are becoming a little incontinent.

- You've gone off sex. And you may notice that your vagina feels tight or dry.

- You may be highly anxious or depressed sometimes.

- You're more forgetful, or feel that you can't think clearly.

- Your weight changes and you feel bloated.
- You get hot and bothered for no reason at all, or sweat profusely at night.
- There are changes in your hair and skin.
- Your eyes are dry and itchy.
- Your voice changes sometimes or is not as strong as it used to be.
- Your sleep pattern may change.
- You generally feel out of sorts.

These changes could just be to do with getting older, or stress, or the way you live your life, but they are also quite likely to be due to the fact that your body's beginning to change as you go through the menopause. And if you are a person who is expecting to notice a few changes as you approach the average age for the menopause, be prepared for the fact that for some women nothing seems to happen for ages.

Eventually, though, your periods will stop. Up to this time, around this time, and after it, you may experience any of the above, and also be aware of other signs and indicators that your body is changing.

WHEN YOU SHOULD SEEK HELP

Many women say that they hardly notice their menopause. But a lot of women experience varying degrees of discomfort at different stages. This can be managed, lessened and relieved in a variety of ways. Plenty of women cope in their own way, and then find in a few years that the whole process has passed. However, some women need lots of help because they do have a tough time.

There is no need to seek medical help just because you are going through the menopause, but if you are worried, if you bleed a little between periods, if you experience real discomfort and feel that you cannot live your life as you wish, you should seek advice. It is important to remember that the changes you notice may be caused by something other than the menopausal process, and your doctor will be able to advise you about this and do any necessary tests.

CHANGES YOU MAY EXPERIENCE

The following are the most common, and often the most distressing changes that women experience during the menopause process. Potentially you could experience some of them at some stage, to a lesser or greater extent.

Understanding the following sections

Please avoid interpreting the following sections as a catalogue of disasters. These are natural changes that occur as part of a natural process. If you are aware and informed, you can decide how best to manage them – and they *can* be managed.

After each section, suggestions are given for some practical ways to help yourself. These do not include the use of any hormone treatment or complementary therapies, herbs or supplements, because these are mentioned later on in part 3

Changes in periods

Leading up to the menopause, you will probably notice changes in the flow and/or the frequency of your periods. You might find that they are much lighter, or much heavier – or both – and there may be no pattern as to whether one time will be light and another heavy. You may have far fewer periods than you used to, or the frequency could remain the same. They might gradually peter out over time, or just stop. So it could well be that your menstrual cycle becomes really unpredictable, and if you have been used to being as regular as clockwork, this can be very disconcerting. One thing that can be really alarming is to find that your period is so heavy that you can hardly stem the flow. If this continues on a regular basis, it may be a good idea to talk to your doctor, because there could be a medical reason for this. But really heavy periods do happen every now and then. It's all part of the process.

What you can do to help yourself

- Avoid the temptation to bulk-buy extra-super-strength tampons and pads. If you do, you can bet that your periods will never again be as heavy, or even stop altogether. The vast amount that you bought will probably stay there, unopened, just in case, for years. And then, when you are post-menopausal, you will probably throw them out.

- Wear dark-coloured skirts or trousers if you know you are going to have a period. At least if it's heavy and you leak, it will be less conspicuous.

- Keep plenty of pads and tampons nearby – in your desk, bag, wherever. You really don't know when you might need them.

- After a very heavy period, rest if you can. Give your body time to restore and replenish itself.

> 66 I did consider buying incontinence pads, but I never needed to. I wore super plus tampons and a big pad. I had to run to the loo fast sometimes though. It can catch you unawares. But you live with it. You can do things like take a spare pair of knickers with you, and wear a full skirt. And you don't sit down. At least that way, if you do flood, you run to the loo and it hasn't marked your skirt. 99
>
> Anna, 63

Hot flush (or flash)

A hot flush is usually the body's reaction to something, and men get them too, sometimes. So, for example, if you eat a hot chili, you may get a hot flush. But at the menopause there is rarely an obvious trigger. There is no definitive reason why these occur at the menopause, but it is likely to be linked to a change in the temperature-controlling part of your brain, in other words the hypothalamus reacting to signals from hormones.

> 66 You might be chatting sociably with friends, and suddenly you notice that they're all flapping their hands at their faces. You're all sitting there like a bunch of chickens – all flapping away. You hardly notice that you're doing it because it's such a habit. All clutching at your clothes to try and flap some cool air in. And all of you are bright red in the face. 99
>
> Sally, 58

Hot flushes range from a sensation of blushing to a feeling of overwhelming heat, and sweating, usually around the upper torso, neck and head. This can lead to feeling flustered, embarrassed and uneasy, especially if you are intensely aware that you look red, patchy and sweaty.

A hot flush can last for a few seconds or for several minutes. You often know that you are about to experience one as you notice your heart beating faster, and a 'hotness' beginning to spread. Sometimes these can be very tricky to manage, especially if you are having them several times a day. In the past you probably had hot flushes to a certain extent just before a period, but for many women they tend to be more common after your periods have stopped altogether.

Hot flushes and make-up

If you like to wear face make-up, it can be devastating when your hot flushes prevent you from doing so. A tip from TV and film make-up artist Gilly Popham is to use a primer first. Some make-ups are designed to be worn in a very hot country where you are likely to sweat. They may also help at menopause if your make-up slithers off your face due to a hot flush. Gilly recommends a mattifier, which will take all of the oil out of your skin, so that it primes it and makes your skin very dry. Wear a very matt make-up, and perhaps try samples until you find a make-up that will work for you. Mattifiers and primers can be bought from most large make-up companies.

Night sweats

This is a hot flush which happens during sleep. It may be quite mild. You might wake up feeling very hot and sweaty, and need to cool down by kicking off the bedclothes. Or you might wake up in bed drenched with sweat and need to keep changing your nightwear and sheets throughout the night. If you have a partner sleeping next to you, they are most likely to be disturbed and on a prolonged basis this can make for grumpiness and distress all round.

> **❝** I'd throw covers off the bed continually, and it was awful. I gave up all stimulants and hot drinks, because I knew that even a hot cup of tea would bring on a hot flush. And I'd always try to get some wind on my face. In the summer, I had to have the fan on all the time – directly on me in bed. I couldn't wear anything in bed, and I made sure the sheets were cotton to absorb the sweat. But then they'd be drenched anyway, and I'd have to change them. And I had cool showers all the time. I just managed in sensible ways, but there wasn't much more that I could do. **❞**
> Di, 63

What you can do to help yourself

Get checked out by your doctor if your hot flushes are really disrupting your life, just to make sure there is no other reason for them. Certain conditions and medications can trigger them. Also, do consider using complementary therapies. Many women have found these helpful.

Stimulants

It is generally accepted that reducing your caffeine and alcohol intake can reduce your hot flushes. Some women find that if they take less tea, coffee, alcohol and chocolate they are much better. So expect that if you have more caffeine or alcohol one day, you could potentially expect to have a couple of days of hot flushes afterwards.

Some women have found that their hot flushes have reduced when they stopped smoking.

Diet

Some say avoid hot, spicy food. There is a chemical (capsaicin) in cayenne pepper and other peppers that is thought may trigger hot flushes. However, some people find that eating really hot spicy food actually cools them down; and it's interesting that food is often spicy in hot countries.

For some, hot flushes are triggered by eating hot (in terms of temperature) food, especially in the evening. (See chapter 11 for more on food and nutrition.)

Drink plenty of water, as cool as possible, throughout the day. It may be an idea to have an ice-cold drink by your bed – in a Thermos flask perhaps.

Clothing

Wear layers of cotton or moisture-absorbing fabric. Then you can remove layers when you need to, to help you cool down. Avoid wearing tight clothes, especially around your neck.

Sleep

You may find a sheet is better than a duvet in bed, but at least with a duvet you can stick limbs out, and often throw the whole thing off yourself without disrupting a sleeping partner too much.

A hot water bottle filled with cold water might bring relief.

Temperature

Keep the air temperature cool – open windows at night, for example, and have an electric fan handy where you are working and by your bed.

You could carry a little battery-driven electric fan in your bag (and spare batteries). This can bring instant relief in uncomfortable moments.

Spraying your face and neck with cool water and letting it dry naturally can help, but this isn't always practical. So put cool water on your wrists and inside elbows, and dab it on your neck and forehead instead. It might help to use aromatherapy oils such as geranium or clary sage like this, too, especially if they are in solid form, such as a solid perfume.

How the professionals stay cool

This tip is used by film and TV make-up artists to help actors cool down when they are very hot: soak a chamois (or other moisture-retaining cloth) in some old-fashioned eau de cologne such as 4711. Wring it out, really shake it and then put it on the back of your neck.

This could work as well for hot flushes as for actors working in hot locations. You could keep a ready-soaked chamois in a make-up purse to carry with you. As you feel the heat rising, take it out, give it a good shake, and put it on the back of your neck (or your forehead if you're not wearing make-up).

Any cheap eau de cologne will do, but not perfume, because that has a different consistency and so doesn't work in the same way.

If you go shopping in hot weather you'll find that large shops and shopping malls are usually air-conditioned so you can wander around for hours in a cool environment, which can be a great relief.

Avoid holidaying where the heat may be relentless – just for the time being.

Invest in a Chillow. This is a thin cooling pad that absorbs your body heat while staying perfectly cold. You fill it with water once, which is fully absorbed, and then it is ready to use. You can put it on top of your pillow, or under your pillowcase, or wherever you wish. I know someone who uses two – she puts one at her head and one round her middle, and now she gets a good night's sleep.

Some women keep one at work to put their feet on, which they find helps them to keep cool.

> **Chillow:**
> www.chillow.co.uk; info@soothsoft.co.uk;
> tel 08700 117174

Using henna for body decoration, especially on the legs and hands, is said to have a cooling effect.

Soothe yourself mentally
Do your best to manage your stress levels. I know this may seem easier said than done, but it is important, and if you take the time to de-stress yourself regularly you will be doing yourself a massive long-term favour. (There's more about relaxation techniques on page 206.)

As your hot flush begins, think of something cooling. It may help to have a picture of this nearby to focus on. For example, a snowy landscape, or a wonderful swimming pool, or a cool marble temple.

A CD of the sound of rain or the ocean could help you feel cooler. You could carry this with you and play it when you are boiling. Give yourself a minute to enjoy it, take deep breaths in, and slow ones out as you let the hot flush pass. In the Royal Gardens in Udaipur, Rajasthan, there is a pool with a central fountain. All around the side are little fountains. The combined effect of these is called 'rain without the clouds'. If you close your eyes and listen, it really does sound like monsoon rain. The sound has an amazingly cooling effect on a very hot day.

Exercise

Any stretching or weight-bearing exercise each day is good, and is thought to cut down the frequency of hot flushes. So walking, swimming, yoga, pilates, tai chi – whatever you fancy. Avoid overdoing it though.

Sex

Some research has shown that women who have sex regularly (once or more a week) have fewer hot flushes.

Disrupted sleep and fatigue

This can be due to a range of things, apart from night sweats. You may be anxious or depressed, and may get off to sleep and then wake in the early hours, churning over thoughts of worry and anxiety for hours on end. Or it may be that you wake up early and can't get back to sleep again. You may long for sleep and rest and feel that you can never get enough.

So you might have a general feeling of tiredness or malaise most of the time. A lot of women going through the menopause describe feeling that they have lost their buzz and vitality. But this isn't the end of the world. It won't last for ever, so take strength from that.

What you can do to help yourself

- Do your best to put the day behind you. Mentally wind down as much as you can. You may find that going through some gentle relaxation exercise before you go to bed helps. If you make an effort to de-stress your mind and body regularly, it becomes a habit and settles nicely into your system.

- If you find yourself awake and you don't want to be, get up and get out of bed. The worst thing is to lie there tossing and turning, or being scared to move in case you waken someone else. If you are anxious, and churning things over in your mind, get out of bed and do something to distract yourself. Make a drink, do anything to break your thought pattern.

- If you usually write with your right hand, write a few lines with the left one, and vice versa. Try drawing circles with one hand, while drawing triangles with the other, and then change over. This sort of thing engages both sides of your brain, which helps to bring your mind into balance.

- Have a book to hand that you really enjoy. Always have something that you *want* to read, that you can lose yourself in. If you wake up, read your book. This is much better than switching on the TV or a film, or going to the computer. The actual act of reading something pleasant and interesting is therapeutic in itself. Eventually, you'll probably find that your eyes are so tired that you can't stay awake.

- Some women find that listening to a story on the radio or an audio book helps them to drift off to sleep. Listening to a relaxation CD can help too. So if you wake up, it may be handy to have this nearby, and an earpiece so that you can listen without disturbing anyone.

- You may find that exercise before you go to bed helps – perhaps a brisk walk or some yoga. If you wake up in the night and decide to exercise, be very gentle with yourself as your mind might be ready but your body may not be – and you could ultimately hurt yourself.

- What you eat and when you eat it can have an effect. The general advice is to have your last meal about two to four hours before you go to bed so that your stomach is not overloaded.

However, some women find that when they wake in the night, a warm drink and a plain biscuit help them to settle. But it's probably best to avoid stimulants like caffeine and alcohol, and heavy foods at night.

- If you feel exhausted because of lack of sleep – you probably are. So rest and relax as much as you are able, because this will do you so much good.

- If you feel that it would help you, change your lifestyle if you can. If, say, you wake at 5am, get up and do the ironing or something, and then go back to bed or have a nap later. There may well be ways that you can adapt and adjust things to suit you right now.

- Most of all, avoid worrying that you aren't getting enough sleep. This will only worry you more. You'll be OK – remember, *this isn't going to last for ever.*

Emotions

The chances are that if you experience your menopause in your late 40s and 50s you will be at a stressful time in your life anyway. You may have a family and elderly parents, all of whom need you in different ways. And you might be at the peak of your career too.

You are probably holding everything together, multi-tasking brilliantly, and coping very well. But if you start experiencing difficulties as you go through the menopause you may feel as if everything comes crashing down, and find it triggers a whole series of events. So you could feel very stressed and exhausted, anxious or depressed.

Your moods may change quickly and you might find yourself tearful at all sorts of times, for all sorts of reasons. You might feel that you are 'falling apart', and worry that you will never feel OK again. On the other hand, you may notice little difference in your emotional well-being at all.

66 A friend of mine cries all the time now. The other day she went into a café and ordered hot chocolate, but they gave her a cappuccino — and she burst into tears. She was so distressed that they came out from behind the counter, helped her into a chair and asked her if there was anyone she'd like them to phone. She said she felt a complete idiot, but she just could not stop crying over something so small.
Rebecca, 43 99

Changes in your emotional state are to be expected, and you've probably got used to this throughout your menstrual life. But women do feel differently about the whole process of menopause, and I think there are three main things to consider here:

● Changing mood states are normal and to be expected. Hormones have an effect on your moods and emotions.

● Depression or high levels of anxiety can sometimes creep in, and you may not have experienced either before.

● You may be saddened by the inevitability that you can no longer conceive. For many women this is a huge issue, and it can take a while to adjust.

❝ I get affected when people make thoughtless statements. Shortly after I had the hysterectomy, a chap who's been good friends with me and my husband for many years said, "Oh look, she's had her engine out.' It was just his way of acknowledging that I'd had major surgery, and I know it wasn't meant unkindly. I laughed it off, but it hurt. **❞**
Trish, 54

❝ I find it hard to come to terms with the fact that I won't be having children again. I do think about that. I would always have liked more children, although I'm too old to cope with a baby now. But there was always that awareness that I could if I wanted to, and now I have to accept the fact that I'm no longer fertile, and I'm getting to the end of the child-rearing phase, and my babies are maturing and will soon be ready to go. I guess it's about coming to terms with all that. **❞**
Clare, 54

Most people feel low sometimes anyway, but this only really becomes depression when it starts to affect your life. Low mood states usually lift, but depression tends to hang around so that you may be aware of a general underlying feeling of helplessness and hopelessness most of the time. And you may also experience quite a lot of anxiety.

Anxiety

Anxiety tends to be a fear of the future, constantly worrying about what may or may not happen. It's fine to be anxious a bit, perhaps if you have something important to do, because it keeps you focused and on your toes. Then, after the event, the mental and physical feelings that go along with anxiety should subside. Typical symptoms are similar to some of the changes that occur during the menopause anyway, such as: feeling very tired and vulnerable, high energy at unusual times, trouble getting to sleep, waking at odd times and not being able to get back to sleep, going over and over things in your mind, weird and vivid dreams, feeling restless and unable to relax, feeling irritable, lack of concentration, feeling 'detached' and spaced out, feeling tense and shaky, feelings of utter and inexplicable fear, joint pains, muscle pains, breathlessness, nausea, feeling faint or dizzy, headaches, palpitations, chest pains and tightness, dry mouth, sweating, skin disorders, stomach pains, and diarrhoea.

If these feelings don't subside, and they become a regular feature in your life, this means that your nervous system is out of balance, and your hormones do have an effect on that.

If high levels of stress and anxiety start to really affect your life, then it is good to do something about it, otherwise the symptoms are unlikely to go away. They just keep building up.

Anxiety attacks
Two of the particularly unpleasant things that can happen as a result of this are that you may have anxiety attacks, or panic attacks. And there is a distinct difference between the two:

- A panic attack comes on very suddenly, and you have no idea why. It can last for any time between several seconds and 10 minutes. Sometimes the symptoms can come in 'waves' for anything up to about two hours. The symptoms can be so intense that you may think you are having a stroke or a heart attack.

- An anxiety attack can come on quickly but it's not usually as severe as a panic attack. You will probably be anxious because of a situation, and will feel the need to escape from it. When you do, you generally feel better.

66 Sometimes I suddenly lose confidence. I don't know what happens, but the thought of driving up the dual carriageway suddenly terrifies me. And I think 'How can I possibly get into this car and drive?' Yet I've driven for years. I'm a good driver, but on some days I just crumble. 99
Jill, 55

66 I've got three teenage boys and a husband. Sometimes I go into the kitchen and I think I'm going to blow up. I feel as if my blood's boiling. I don't know why I react like that now. Mornings are the worst. I go into the kitchen and they're all in there. They all look so big, and seem to fill the place up so much. Even just seeing their shoes by the door – I hate it. There are so many of them –eight shoes lying there. I feel so mean, it never used to bother me. 99
Meg, 52

What you can do to help yourself

- Be gentle with yourself. You are going through a process. It's quite natural for your emotions to be all over the place at this time.

- Learn something of anxiety and depression. This way, you will understand what is happening to you. This is really helpful, because knowledge and understanding take away the fear. When you understand how anxiety attacks and panic attacks come about, you can start to do something about them. There's lots of information about this in my book *How Not To Worry* (White Ladder Press, 2008).

- If you feel that your emotions are getting out of hand, it could be a good idea to seek some help. It's always good to talk to someone about how you feel, rather than bottling it all up.

- Avoid feeling stupid or weak. You are not. You are a woman coping with the changes in the best way that you can. You may feel that your confidence has hit rock bottom – but that's natural. It will come back. Just look after yourself in the meantime, and let things be for now. You can take back your power when you are ready.

- Expect to feel hurt, or misunderstood, sometimes. Other people probably have no idea how you feel because they have their own issues. Look for the positives in any situation, and choose something that pleases you to focus on, so that your negative emotions fade into the background.

- Be with other women when you can. It's amazing how you can support each other.

- Make a point of doing something just for you that is fun and interesting. Things like yoga and tai chi are great for helping you to come back into balance. Or you might like to sing or dance or do something else creative.

● Do some regular exercise that you enjoy. This can give you a real emotional boost and can help you to see things from a wider perspective.

Bouncing

You might like to try this as a way of overcoming a sense of frustration, irritation and general 'fed-upness'.

Buy a small, circular trampoline – a rebounder, or trampette – about one metre in diameter.

Just enjoy jumping up and down on it for a few minutes every now and then. It's great exercise and great fun. It can be quite aerobic, especially if you circle your arms, or do a breaststroke movement as if you're swimming. You can synchronise it with your breathing too.

Place it in front of a mirror – preferably not a full-length one. As you bounce, face the mirror. Think about how fed up/irritated/frustrated you feel as you bounce, or better still, speak your thoughts and feelings out loud. Just notice what happens.

Do you still have those negative feelings now? I bet they've dissolved as you bounced and noticed your reflection bouncing too. Did the expression on your face change? Was your hair flying, and were your earrings bouncing? Did you laugh?

It's good fun to turn around as you bounce on a trampette. The entire environment looks different somehow, and you can face whichever way you like. And why not make a noise as you jump? It'll lift your spirits. When I do this, my family think I'm crazy – but who cares? I'm having fun.

Medical warning: This form of exercise may not be appropriate if you have certain medical conditions, so please check with your doctor first if you think this could apply to you.

Trampettes are pretty good for jogging too. In fact, if you look on the internet, you'll find a range of exercises that you can do. Put 'trampette' or 'rebounder' into a search engine.

Weight gain

As your hormone levels change, so does your metabolism, so you may well burn off calories at a slower rate. Therefore you may store more fat. Also, the fat is redistributed and tends to increase around your waist, so you might find that your shape changes, which can make you feel that you have 'put on weight'.

> **66** I was always tiny, but I was mortified when I couldn't fasten my trousers. And I felt that my face looked fatter. So I had to buy new clothes. I kept the old ones though and two years later I could wear them again easily.
> Helen, 57 **99**

What you can do to help yourself
- Avoid worrying about this, because it may all change again.
- Wear clothes that fit. If your clothes are too tight you will not look and feel your best.
- Avoid the urge to get rid of all your smaller-size clothes. You will probably fit into them perfectly in a few months.
- Drink plenty of water to keep your system hydrated and therefore working as well as it can.
- Exercise – walking will do, or you could join a belly dancing class or use a hula hoop to whittle away the centimetres. If you

want to use a hula hoop, it's best to get one that is weighted properly, otherwise it won't stay in place very well as you swivel your hips.

Tender breasts

You may find that your breasts are sore and tender due to the fluctuating hormone levels in your body. Perhaps they feel tight or ache, and they may be swollen. This can happen every so often, and it can affect one or both breasts. On the other hand you may have tender breasts most of the time at some stage or other during the menopause. You may also be aware of tiny lumps. Avoid fretting about this. This is most likely to be due to the hormonal changes, but it is worth talking to the doctor just to eliminate any other causes for these symptoms.

What you can do to help yourself

- It may help to limit your intake of caffeine and salt.

- Buy a bra that 'protects' your breasts whilst they are uncomfortable. So possibly one with some padding, or under-wiring, and one that 'holds' you in place comfortably, with strong new straps, as opposed to limp, old ones.

- Some women find that the Chillow pad (see **hot flushes**, above) is a comfort at night.

Headaches and migraines

You may get headaches. Changes in hormone levels can trigger headaches and migraines in some women. I remember that I got the most terrible migraine on two occasions in my mid-40s – something I have never experienced before or since. On reflection, I am sure it was to do with the early stages of menopause because it tied in with other relevant factors at the time.

On the other hand, if you are usually prone to headaches and migraines, you may find they diminish and disappear as you go through menopause.

What you can do to help yourself

- Keep your blood sugar levels up and so avoid skipping meals.

- Take the time to de-stress each day by being completely silent for a few minutes, or follow a technique such as that mentioned on page 206.

- Avoid caffeine and other migraine-inducing foods such as cheese and chocolate.

- Some women find that placing their head on something cool such as the Chillow pad helps.

Aches and pains

Aches and pains are quite common, especially in your lower back, knees, feet, ankles, wrists and shoulders. You may worry that you have the onset of a condition such as arthritis. While this may be possible, your discomfort is more likely to be due to tension and posture, exacerbated by the fluctuation in hormone levels. Eventually it will pass, and there are things that you can do to help yourself.

66 In the last year-and-a-half I've noticed lots of joint aches in my shoulders, elbows and wrists, and knees. I think some of this is tension, but I walk a lot now, and do tai chi. I sleep better since I've been doing that too.

Nikki, 56 99

66 First thing in the morning I could hardly get out of bed. My lower back, heels and legs ached so much. It took me a while to straighten up, and I felt like an old woman. I had some Alexander Technique lessons and they really sorted me out. **99**
Jennie, 48

Poor posture is responsible for lots of aches and pains, and tension may cause you to hold yourself in a less than helpful way.

What you can do to help yourself

- De-stress your body daily with a relaxation technique (see page 206).

- Treat yourself to some Alexander Technique lessons (see page 170) which will help you to let go of unhelpful postural and movement habits and replace them with much better ones.

- Check out your footwear. Your feet should be planted firmly and broadly on the ground, not tottering on tiptoes and balancing on spiky heels.

- Check your shoulders for tension regularly, and release them. Just let them drop. You could also raise them to your ears first, and then let them drop; and rotate them slowly from time to time. It's amazing how much tension you can carry in your shoulders, when you are sitting or standing.

Mental functioning

You may notice that you are forgetful or can't concentrate, or feel generally more muddled than you used to. You probably do bizarre things sometimes, such as write down someone's phone number and then throw it away, or put teaspoons in the rubbish bin with the teabag.

Perhaps you watch and enjoy a film and then can't remember what it was about. This is far more likely to be due to your hormonal activity than the development of a deteriorating mental condition. I know that this can be a niggling worry for a lot of women as they get older, especially if there is a history of something such as Alzheimer's disease in your family.

> I went to work wearing a suit and odd shoes. One was blue and one was black. I can't believe I did that. I'm so particular – I would never have done that before.
> Les, 48

You may also be aware that you feel detached from everyone and everything, as if you are going around in a fog. Or you might feel as if you are detached from yourself – as if you are watching yourself from outside. These are common symptoms of anxiety, and also are quite likely to be connected to hormones fluctuating.

> I drove through red traffic lights once. I thought red meant 'go', which was dreadful because I know red means 'stop'.
> Nora, 50

> I made a mental note of where I'd parked the car, but when I came out of the precinct I couldn't remember where it was. I pushed a full

shopping trolley through acres of busy car park to try and find it, and after 20 minutes I was nearly in tears. Every other car seemed to be the same colour and shape as mine. Eventually I just stumbled across it, but I don't remember parking there at all. I felt so stupid. What's even worse was that a few weeks later I did exactly the same thing.

Fiona, 56

99

What you can do to help yourself

- Exercise your brain by challenging yourself. So do something new, different and fun that makes you focus and think in a different way. This could be studying something, or doing crosswords, or meeting new groups of people so that the interaction is new and fresh and interesting. This will help you to feel that you are taking control and are doing the best that you can.

- Make lists if you need to, and write things down. It can be a good idea to carry a small spiral-bound notebook with you – that way, you can tear pages out when you're finished with them. The advantage of having one book instead of various bits of paper is that you will get into the habit of using it and everything will be written in one place.

- If your mobile phone has a voice recording facility, use it. I often just record the name of the street where I have parked and a landmark, or even which floor I'm on in a multi-storey car park. Otherwise, just like Fiona, I get immersed in whatever I'm doing, and can end up wandering around for ages looking for my car.

- Know and accept that you are not stupid or foolish. This happens to most women, and it's part of the process of the menopause. So just accept that. It's OK, and it really doesn't last for ever.

- Avoid letting any unkind remarks (even those that are said unintentionally) get you down. When you are worried about the state of your mind, any reference to it, or joke made about it, can send your confidence crashing and can really hurt you. But other people are unlikely to know how vulnerable and worried you might be. I had a client whose husband teased her about her forgetfulness quite often. He did it affectionately, but she hated it, especially when he did it in front of others. She found that the best way to deal with it was to smile sweetly and agree with him. He soon stopped, because he didn't know how to respond to her reaction.

- Eat good nutritious food, including wholegrains, fruit and vegetables.

- Exercise your body, and de-stress yourself daily, so that you can think in a calm, clear way.

- Sleep well (if you can). If waking at night is an issue, then learning to relax your body thoroughly is doubly important. (See page 206 for a relaxation technique.)

66 Sometimes I feel as if there's too much information going into too small a brain.
Paula, 56 99

Vaginal changes

The whole subject of your vagina and sex can be perplexing and worrying as you go through the menopause. You may wonder why you are prone to infections, or why sex might be uncomfortable or, indeed, why you have lost interest in the whole thing.

As your sex hormone levels fall, the vaginal walls become less elastic and thinner. Your vagina becomes shorter, and your natural lubricating solutions become more watery, so you can feel dry and sore, or itchy. Therefore, sexual intercourse may be awkward or painful, and you may notice changes in your vaginal discharge. Also, the genital tissue around your vagina becomes thinner.

All this is a perfectly natural state of affairs, but the whole process has been given the rather unfortunate label of 'atrophy of the vagina and labia'. Atrophy means 'wither', 'shrivel' and 'waste away' – hardly a boost to a woman's confidence.

What you can do to help yourself

- Keep your vagina lubricated to be more comfortable and to help with the mechanics of sex. It's best to seek advice from a health practitioner about what to use, as there is a range of products available and they may not all be suitable for you.

- Do regular pelvic floor exercises as mentioned on page 113, to keep everything in best working order. The effect of these can also increase sexual pleasure.

- Avoid using soap or deodorant around your genitals. If you wear panty liners, wear ones that are unscented.

- Wear cotton underwear so that the genital area can 'breathe'.

- Avoid wearing underwear, tights or trousers that are too tight.

Interest in sex

Many women find that they take a great deal longer to become sexually aroused at menopause, and some lose interest in sex altogether. Obviously this is quite a delicate area to consider, and there are products and lubricating creams to make the physical side of sex easier.

But the whole mental and emotional side is something else. To be honest, if you are exhausted, waking up repeatedly at night (probably drenched with sweat), unable to get back to sleep afterwards, and feeling generally grumpy and emotional; if you feel your confidence dwindles as you lose track of what you are saying mid-sentence, and forget things as soon as you think of them; if you have aches and pains, and maybe a bladder infection as well; if your skin is dry and you have put on weight – well, is it any wonder that you may not feel like having sex?

And is it any wonder that your partner may be perplexed and grumpy as they too wake up several times each night in your drenched bed?

> ❝ The desire is there, but it takes me forever to climax now. I 've asked for Viagra, but the doctor won 't prescribe it for me.
> Stella, 56 ❞

> ❝ I 've lost interest in sex completely really. I 'd far rather go to bed and read my book. My husband 's very understanding, but it 's not fair on him.
> Connie, 51 ❞

There is nothing wrong or 'odd' here - it's just a question of adjustment, and your discomfort will not last for ever.

> **"** A lot of women say that they've lost libido, but it doesn't bother them, and they're not particularly worried about it. They are far more worried about how it affects their partner. Loss of libido is never just one thing. There are usually multi-factors — all the physical symptoms like hot flushes, vaginal dryness and not sleeping. And then the lifestyle and emotional situations — things like teenagers having been away at university and suddenly pitching up at home again, caring for your parents, changes in jobs, changes in your partner's situation, maybe divorce — there's a whole range of things that, combined, affect libido. Once these things are resolved or managed, often your libido comes back. And if you can help to reduce the menopausal symptoms, then hopefully that will have a knock-on effect on libido.
>
> Sometimes, if a woman has had her ovaries removed, a lack of libido can be due to the drop in testosterone, (the ovaries produce a small amount of testosterone). This drop is not significant for some women, but for others it's very important for libido and energy levels. Testosterone replacement can be given to balance this.
>
> Amanda Hillard, clinical nurse specialist who runs a menopause clinic **"**

What you can do to help yourself
- Talk about how you feel with your sexual partner. This is the most important thing to do, because without communication you are stumped. Neither of you will know how the other thinks

or feels – you can only guess. If you are able to communicate, then you can plan a way forward – together.

- Do what you can to stay in good health, so eat well and exercise moderately. Relax and de-stress as often as you can.

- Avoid feeling less of a woman because you have less interest in sex than you used to have.

- Seek professional help if you wish, and avoid being embarrassed about the fact that you are doing so.

Sleeping arrangements

I reckon many double beds get thrown on the tip around the time of a woman's menopause. Many couples find it far less hassle to sleep separately, either in the same room in separate beds, or in different rooms.

66 For years and years we've slept with two single beds put together so that I don't disturb my husband. We make it up as a double, so we manage with one duvet, because neither of us tosses and turns that much, but it's the mattress moving that disturbs him. My husband has always been a light sleeper. And I used to sleep brilliantly before the menopause. I never woke in the night at all then.
Di, 63 **99**

- It doesn't matter how many times you wriggle, twitch, move, turn over, get up – it is far less likely to disturb your partner than if you share the same mattress.

- You let go of the whole 'If I move I'll disturb them' thing, so you are automatically less stressed.

- If you wake up in a bed drenched with sweat, you can change it without disturbing your partner.

- You can each have a covering that suits you – if you want a sheet you can have it, and your partner can have a 50 tog quilt if they wish.

- If you are in separate rooms you won't be able to hear each other snoring.

This doesn't mean that you can't cuddle or have sex – it's just a sleeping arrangement. I knew a couple who had a double bed, with a single bed next to it so that one of them could roll into the single bed any time they felt the need.

66 I wake up in the night far more than I used to. I don't sleep in the same bed as my husband any more, because he's such a light sleeper. I used to toss and turn, worrying that I was keeping him awake, and keeping him from the best sleep he could have that night, so I'd be lying there very still, while I was trying to sleep – which just made me worse.

Annette, 55 99

Of course you may want to stay in the same bed as each other no matter what. And it may be that your partner sleeps very soundly and is rarely disturbed. The key thing is to do whatever works for you.

Some people assume that there must be something wrong with a relationship if they discover that partners are sleeping separately. And I've known partners themselves to be quite embarrassed by the fact that they are doing so. But why? OK, human beings have sex and procreate, but whoever said that they had to spend the whole night together in the same bed?

Mandi

*For **Mandi**, 52, overwhelming tiredness has been a real issue, and she has learnt to deal with that by listening to her body and responding accordingly. She has a positive and focused approach to the menopause.*

"There have been times when I haven't had a period for about four or five months, but then they usually start again with a vengeance. And at other times I've had very heavy periods and then have missed a couple after that.

"When I have a hot flush I experience an overwhelming heat - mainly around my head, and no-where else. I get extremely tired. I find that I do need far more sleep than I used to. If I have a couple of late nights, I have to have a night where I go to bed early and sleep for 14 hours or so. The tiredness is a real issue for me. It's overwhelming – like when I was pregnant. I can hardly get out of bed. I go to the gym two or three times a week. If I don't do that, I do find I'm much more tired.

"I am aware that I am far less tolerant of people when I think they're being unfair or unreasonable.

"I don't know much about HRT. I think if I was having the heavy periods that I was prone to a few years ago, I might have to consider some medication because I know it's not a good idea to lose too much blood. But the menopause is going to happen whether you like it or not, so you might as well let it happen naturally. If you're too poorly to work - you're too poorly to work. I don't particularly want to work anyway now, and maybe that's part of it. I've never felt that I didn't want to work before. So maybe this is the menopause telling my body to slow down, and just let it happen naturally. I feel quite positive about the whole thing anyway."

Agatha

Agatha *is 54 and happy to look forward to the next phase of her life. She's had to adapt and make changes in order to manage her menopause, particularly her hot flushes.*

"My periods started becoming irregular about four years ago. I was going without one for three or four months and really worried I might be pregnant. But I haven't had a period for two-and-a-half years now.

"Then I started to get hot flushes. I'd feel my cheeks burning first, and the sweat would pour off my face. When we were out, if I had a hot flush – usually when having dinner in the evening - I'd have to go outside or open a window. I'd be sweating, wet through and feel so embarrassed, and that made me irritable. We'd have to go home early, because I was so sick of it. Sometimes I can get three or four a day, and sometimes I go for days without any at all. So they're not regular. And I've gone weeks and not had one, and then they come back with a vengeance.

"They can happen day or night. At night I have to throw the covers off and open windows. My nightdress is soaked - actually I've had to stop wearing nightclothes. But it's not as bad as it used to be. Everything in bed used to be absolutely drenched. I used to lie on towels, which soaked the sweat up.

"The doctor suggested HRT – but I wasn't sure. I think that the menopause is a natural thing, so I thought I'd try and sort it out myself if I could. The doctor suggested that I don't drink tea or coffee after lunchtime, and I've noticed that if I have a coffee after that, I start sweating and then I can't sleep at night, and it's worse than ever. The same applies to alcohol. So now I drink a lot of water.

"The doctor also noticed that I'd put on a lot of weight. I used to horse ride, but then I stopped three years ago, after my sister-in-law had a bad riding accident. Now I walk, and I do water aerobics. It's easier than ordinary aerobics, and when you get hot, you don't notice the sweat as much. So I've lost weight again, although I don't eat less.

"But I've noticed a couple of things: my nails are really brittle and break easily now, and I now really hate going to have cervical smears. I find it more unpleasant every time I go now. It never used to worry me when I was younger, and when I had the children it was all par for the course. But now I find it extremely unpleasant and quite painful. I feel as though something has invaded my body.

"My general feeling about the menopause is that I'm into the next phase of my life now, and I'm very happy with that. I'm happy with the fact that my daughters are adults now, and I certainly don't want any more children. The menopause has been a damn nuisance more than anything, but I accept that it's part of a process. I just want it to finish altogether now."

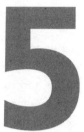

Changes during the menopause

Some of the changes listed below may or may not be directly connected to the menopause, but they probably are indicators of the hormonal activity taking place. In many ways, no-one really knows. Research and statistics cannot hope to take into account *every* woman, or *every* change that she experiences.

If you are noticing changes in yourself and wonder if it could be to do with the menopause, then the chances are that it is. It may also be age-related, lifestyle-related, stress-related, or something else, and if you are concerned do visit the doctor and get checked out. But bear in mind that the process of the menopause takes some time. The changes you notice at the very start may be totally different from those you experience later on. Some of these changes are:

Gum disease

It's important to look after your teeth and gums because the decrease in oestrogen affects your gums, and of course the ageing process makes a difference too. This is more important than you may realise, as gum disease can ultimately affect your heart as the infected bacteria get into your blood. During the menopause, because of the hormone levels changing, the gums are hypersensitive and they react more violently to any plaque or bacteria that you leave in your mouth.

How they react varies from person to person. If your gums are basically healthy to start with, they can cope, although at certain times in the month they may get slightly more irritated. But if you have gums that are not healthy to start with, then this just exacerbates everything.

Gum disease, commonly known as gingivitis, is caused by the build-up of bacteria and plaque between your gums and teeth. So you may have bleeding round your teeth and gums, and bad breath. Your gums probably also look red, when they should be pink. At the same time, you may find that there is some bone loss around your teeth and jaw, so that your teeth are in danger of eventually falling out.

What you can do to help yourself

- Have regular dental check-ups. If you have some gum disease you will probably be recommended to a dental hygienist who will thoroughly clean your teeth and show you how to look after them really well. If you follow their advice, your gums should shrink back to being strong and healthy again.

- If you have to pay for dental treatment, it may well be worth looking into taking out a dental care plan, because the extra visits to a hygienist can all mount up.

Bloating, water retention and wind

Oestrogen affects water retention. As the level of oestrogen rises you tend to retain more fluid, which is why so many people feel bloated just before a period. As hormone levels change so much during the menopause, it is quite common to feel bloated. Also, many people seem to have more intestinal gas around this time, and it is thought that change in hormone levels affect this too. There can be many other reasons though, including your diet and certain medical conditions. But the need to fart or burp regularly is not a particularly attractive characteristic, and there are things that you can do to alleviate this.

What you can do to help yourself

- Many practitioners would suggest monitoring your diet in the first instance, because it may be that some foods affect you more than others, such as wheat, or sugar. You may not tolerate certain foods as well as you used to, but this can change. For instance, you may find that dried fruit affects your digestion *at the moment,* so leaving it out of your diet for a few weeks could make all the difference. Keep a food journal for a while so that you can monitor this.

- Drink plenty of water. This helps to flush out the system.

Changes in skin

You tend to lose some skin protein (collagen) around the time of the menopause because oestrogen stimulates the production of collagen. So as the oestrogen levels diminish, so too does the collagen. This can make the skin drier, thinner, and more likely to itch. Sometimes you may find that you have really itchy patches on your body, which are annoying and uncomfortable. And you may get spots.

What you can do to help yourself

- Eat good, nutritious food. Keep to a balanced diet and avoid junk food.

- Avoid smoking and too much alcohol or caffeine. Smoking in particular is known to age the skin.

- Get plenty of exercise and fresh air.

- Drink lots of water. It's amazing how keeping hydrated can 'plump' up your skin, and help you to look younger in a very short space of time.

- Rest and de-stress as much as you can.

- Keep to a good daily skin care routine avoiding perfumed chemicals, and moisturise wherever your skin feels dry.

Brittle nails

This is very common, and it is thought that the most likely cause of dry, brittle or weak nails in women of menopausal age is the fluctuating levels of oestrogen, although a change in nail quality could be indicative of an illness or deficiency of some kind. And the skin around the nails can be very painful if it is full of little cuts.

What you can do to help yourself

- Avoid putting your hands in water as much as you can. Wear rubber gloves whenever you do any chores, and when your hands are in water, such as when washing up. This protects your nails and the skin around them from being bombarded with chemicals, and also keeps them out of the water.

- Invest in a really good hand cream. Ones containing tea tree oil can be good.

- As soon as you have a taste of cold weather and wind, wear gloves when outside.

- Briskly rub the nails of one hand against those of the other as often as possible. This improves circulation and can be a good toner generally.

- A dietary supplement may help you.

Changes in hair

You may find that your hair becomes thinner, and you lose some, or it may become coarser in texture. You might have less underarm and pubic hair, but you might have more hair on your face. This is all to do with your hormone levels changing, and the balance shifting. Extra facial hair is caused by the change in the level of the male sex hormone, testosterone.

❝ My hair used to be really thick. Now I only have about a third of what I used to have. I know another woman who used to have thick, voluptuous curls when she was younger, and now she has really thin, fine hair. She said she'd thought she was going bald.
Angela, 54 **❞**

❝ When my daughter was 10 she pointed at my face and said accusingly, 'Er – yuk! Witches have those.' I rushed to the mirror. There, sprouting determinedly from a mole on my chin, was a single sprout of hair. I was 45.
Caroline, 53 **❞**

What you can do to help yourself

- Choose a style that suits the texture of your hair and keep to a good hair-care routine avoiding perfumed chemicals.

- Eat good, nutritious food. Keep to a balanced diet and avoid junk food.

- Avoid smoking, too much alcohol or caffeine.

- Get plenty of exercise and fresh air.

- Drink lots of water.

- Rest and de-stress as much as you can.

Changes in body odour

There may be all sorts of reasons for changes in your body odour. Your diet, for example. But it is thought that hormonal changes affect body odour too, and it may be linked to the amount that you sweat. Some women appear to have little body odour, and for some it can be devastating to realise that for the first time in their lives they have acquired 'an aroma'.

What you can do to help yourself

Personal hygiene is obviously important, but avoid over-washing and bathing or using strongly scented soaps or deodorants. These can irritate the natural balance of the secretions on your skin. The best thing to do is to seek advice, as there are products and therapies that can help. For example, Helena (below) found that Chinese medicine and acupuncture helped her.

" For the first time ever, I was aware of my own smell at menopause. Especially with hot flushes. It worried me. I don't want to smell rancid. Chinese medicine helped. I had acupuncture,

and herbs which I had to boil up into tea. I'm
sure it's gone now. I certainly feel much better
about it.

99

Helena, 50

Dry eyes

You may be aware of dry eyes to a greater or lesser degree during
the menopause process. If your eyes feel hot, gritty and itchy
it may be due to the fact that you are not producing enough
tears, and/or a lack of oil in the inner eyelids. Hormones play an
important role in the lubrication of your eyes, and some studies
have shown that the sex hormones may be directly linked to
the production of tears, so it is likely that the change in these
hormone levels will affect the moistness of your eyes.

66 I got dry eyes after the menopause. It was
dreadful. I thought it was because I wasn't
sleeping. But the doctor said it was to do with the
tear ducts, and that I'd always have the problem
so I'd have to use eye drops. But I became
allergic to the drops.

I now use something called Clarymist which is a
fine spray which you spray onto closed eyes and
it's absorbed through the eyelids. It helps to
normalise the lipid layer on the eye which helps to
retain the moisture in your eyes. I couldn't do
without it now — it has really helped me. I still
probably have dry eyes but it just stops them
drying out even more. You can buy it in the major

chemists and some supermarkets now, but at first I had to send off for it.

And since I've had the allergy with my eyes I can't use any cosmetics whatsoever. I always used to wear eye make-up. But I must say, when I stopped using it nobody said anything, so it couldn't have made a remarkable difference. Personally, I feel I need eye make up because I know what I looked like with it. But I've just got used to not using it. I think you just have to accept it really. It's better than going round with your eyes smarting.

Di, 63

Clarymist:
www.clarymist.co.uk; tel 08450 60 60 70

Although it is thought that there is no direct link between the menopause and eyesight, your eyes do change with age. Dry eyes can affect your vision, because it may become blurred, and you might find that your eyes are extra sensitive to light.

As a general point, if you work at a computer, avoid sitting staring at it for more than 20 minutes at a time. As a writer I know how easy it is to become absorbed in what I'm doing and the time flies by. Quite often I set an alarm to remind me. The idea is to work for 20 minutes, then look at something in the distance for at least 20 seconds. This helps you to avoid unnecessary eyestrain, and probably headaches too.

Changes to your voice

You may be aware that your voice becomes deeper, or more hoarse or husky as you progress through menopause. This is usually because the vocal cords thicken. (Remember that sex hormones have an effect on the voice at puberty, so it makes perfect sense that they have an effect at the time of the menopause too.) But it is also important to understand that any anxiety and emotional change affects your voice, as do tiredness and illness. If you are aware that you sound different, you may lose confidence a bit, but there are things that you can do which will help you to feel more confident when you speak.

What you can do to help yourself

- If you are concerned that there may be something wrong with your voice, it would be a good idea to see the doctor in the first instance.

- Drink lots of water throughout the day to keep your voice hydrated.

- Relax and de-stress your body each day if you can. This will have a really beneficial effect on your voice.

- Contact the wonderful Voice Care Network UK, which helps people to keep their voices healthy and to communicate effectively. VCN will be able to give you advice, and lead you to a voice therapist or coach should you need one. They also offer workshops which will show you how to use your voice without straining it. Many women, such as teachers, who have to use their voices a great deal in their work have found these really useful.

Voice Care:
www.voicecare.org.uk; info@voicecare.org.uk; tel 01926 864000

The following are some other issues that may concern you. They can occur at any time.

Yeast infections

The most common of these is vaginal thrush, which is a yeast infection caused by the candida albicans fungus that lives in the gut. Candida albicans itself is thought to be harmless, but when it multiplies it can cause havoc in your system. Infections usually start in the vagina or mouth.

Vaginal thrush usually manifests as itching, burning and soreness of the vagina, along with a thick, creamy, odourless discharge. Many women experience vaginal thrush, and although it usually affects women in their 30s and 40s, and those who are pregnant, it can occur later on. Research has shown that candida albicans thrives on progesterone, which may be why some women are prone to thrush just before a period.

If you have thrush, your symptoms may be quite mild; on the other hand the whole thrush experience can make you feel really fed up. It can be far more debilitating than many people realise. Thrush can also recur. Medically it can be treated with anti-fungal medicine, cream or pessaries, and many women have found that complementary therapies have helped to relieve and cure them of recurring thrush.

Thrush and another yeast infection, candida, tend to be lumped together, but there is a difference. Candida is when the bacteria multiply so much that they get into your whole system through the intestinal wall. Not everyone who has candida has thrush, although many people do, as thrush is just one of the symptoms of candida. Both men and women can experience candida, but it is more common among women.

It is thought that some women may be more prone to candida than others, for example if they are diabetic, or have a weak immune system. Hormonal changes, stress and the use of various medications are also thought to have an effect.

Claire is a young woman who has had candida since she was 14. She has type 1 diabetes, which means that she is insulin-dependent so has to inject herself. Though she has no experience of menopause yet, her story is interesting, and her comments below give a sense of the impact that candida can have. You can read a fuller version of Claire's story on page 102.

" Candida took absolute control of my whole body. It started as thrush, and I was very tired and depressed. I couldn't sleep properly and I became extremely forgetful. I started to get really bad food cravings to the point that I was actually binge-eating all sorts of rubbish. As someone with diabetes, I would never usually do that. I have to be very careful especially around the time of my period, when the hormonal fluctuation affects my blood sugar levels. I was prescribed antibiotics but they made it worse as they depleted all the good bacteria in my gut. I've learnt that the most important thing is to cut out sugar from my diet in every form, including fruit unfortunately, because that makes it much worse. Food combining is really important because if you're eating fruit after a meal, for example, it just ferments in the stomach on top of the carbohydrates you've eaten – and the candida loves that. And you need to replace the good bacteria in your system, and herbs and supplements can help with that. But there might be other things to do with your immune system that need sorting out as well. You have to treat the cause, not the symptoms.

Claire, 28

99

Claire Short

Claire Short is a nutritional adviser and is happy to assist anyone with candida issues: cshort124@googlemail.com

National Candida Society: www.candida-society.org

What you can do to help yourself

- Drink lots of water to keep your system flushed out.

- Eat plain, live, unsweetened yoghurt, especially if you are taking antibiotics as well. The bacteria in the yoghurt help to balance the natural PH level in the body, which helps to keep the yeast under control.

- You can also insert yoghurt into the vagina on a tampon, which may help to balance the vaginal PH level. You could try this every night for a week or so.

- Some women have found that inserting a peeled clove of garlic wrapped in muslin into the vagina helps – but it stinks.

- Some women find tea tree oil is useful, either on a tampon or diluted with water to bathe the vaginal area. This can sting a bit, but the stinging wears off.

- Exercise as usual to keep everything working as well as it can, and eat good, nutritious food – but you may need to review your diet because some foodstuffs may be exacerbating the issue. It may be helpful to take advice about this, especially if you find the yeast infection recurs.

- Avoid using soap or deodorant around your genital area. If you wear panty liners, wear ones that are unscented.

- Avoid leaving tampons and contraceptive sponges, caps or diaphragms in place for too long.

- Wear cotton underwear so that the genital area can 'breathe'.

- Avoid wearing underwear, tights or trousers that are too tight.

- Wipe from front to back when you go to the toilet to avoid transferring bacteria.

Fibroids

Fibroids are growths in the womb. They are round lumps which may be tiny, or they may grow large. Many women have them, although it's not known why. They tend to occur prior to the menopause, because they grow with high levels of oestrogen. Then usually after the menopause, when the oestrogen level drops, they shrink. But sometimes they appear later on as well.

You may not know that you have fibroids if they don't bother you at all – and that's fine. On the other hand, they may cause you much distress, such as pain in your abdomen, bloating, heavy periods, pain when urinating or emptying your bowels, infertility, or miscarriage. Occasionally, a fibroid may be cancerous.

If necessary, you may have to have an operation to remove your fibroids, but in many cases medication suffices.

Ovarian cyst

This is a cyst that grows inside an ovary. A cyst is a sac that is filled with fluid, which can vary in consistency from watery to fairly solid. They are very common, vary in size, are usually painless and last for a few weeks. But if they grow too large they can cause problems, which you could confuse with the changes that you notice through your menopause. For example, they may affect your hormones, and you might get pains and changes in your periods. You may wonder if you have a bladder infection. Just occasionally, a cyst may be an indication of ovarian cancer.

If you are concerned, your doctor can check you physically and, if necessary, refer you for a scan. If you are post-menopausal you will be monitored quite carefully with scans and blood tests just to make sure that there are no malignancies there.

> An ovarian cyst is caused by the body trying to cleanse itself of poisons. The body can't get rid of the poisons, so it creates these sacs to put the poison in. By cleansing the body, balancing your hormones and having high fibre in your diet, you can help your body rid itself of these cysts. The body finds it very difficult to produce eggs when it is covered in cysts. So, if you balance the body with supplements, and let it cleanse itself, you can help your body return to good health.
>
> Dinah Smith, natural health adviser

Angela

Angela, *54, is delighted to be post-menopausal now. However, she has high blood pressure and has been losing her hair for the past seven years.*

"I'm fiery and hot-tempered anyway, and used to have terrible mood swings before a period, so I can't say I've noticed the menopause that much. Perhaps a more placid person would notice more if they got moody or irritable.

"My periods were never regular, and they were terrible when I was a teenager. They were very erratic, and they'd last for about 10 days and be very painful. When I was about 47 they became very scanty and started to peter out, and by the time I was 50 they'd stopped.

"I got hot flushes for a couple of years, but they weren't bad at all. Just like a feeling of heat passing through my entire body and limbs, but not my face. I don't have any sexual interest at all, and I'm not bothered about that. I had spates of headaches for about six weeks at a time, and I still get those.

"But my hair is falling out – I've been losing hair since I was 47. Every time I brush my hair there's so much in the brush. My hair used to be really thick; now I only have about a third of what I used to have. I think that all of this could be exacerbated by anger and anxiety, because my current personal circumstances are not helpful.

"But I've no emotional feelings about the menopause. It was wonderful to think that I couldn't conceive any more. Who wants to conceive at 50 anyway? Having two children was plenty for me, and I have a grandchild to enjoy now. I'd rather have my hair back than be able to conceive."

Claire

Claire, 28, has had candida since she was 14.

"Candida albicans is the bacteria that lives in the gut, and that's normally where it starts. So most women will find that they'll get vaginal yeast infections first, and also in the mouth. You might end up with a white film on your tongue or in the corners of your mouth and cracked lips. Then the candida penetrates through your gut. This is when people get leaky gut syndrome – it gets into your bloodstream, and that's when it starts to affect the organs and the brain. You can find that you develop food allergies, and you might feel bloated, or have diarrhoea or constipation. Candida really does affect everything dramatically.

"I've had candida on and off since I was about 14, but more severely and constantly for the last two years. I started off getting thrush. It just wouldn't go away. Then I started getting very tired, very depressed and stressed, and blamed it on all sort of other things, for example my diabetes.

"But then I read lots of books about candida and I realised that it might be that. But the doctor told me that there was no such thing, and that I had thrush. I was given antibiotics to get rid of it. But these made it worse, because they depleted all the good bacteria. It had actually got into my whole system. It was affecting my brain, my sleep patterns, and how much energy I had. I'd forget things, and I'd forget whole conversations. I thought I must be going crazy. I'd forget things that happened not just a month, week or day ago, but even after an hour.

"I started to get really bad food cravings to the point that I was actually binge eating all sorts of rubbish. As someone with diabetes, I would never usually do that. I'd find myself in the shop in the queue with a huge bar of chocolate. By the time I'd got home I'd have eaten the lot. With diabetes, you're prone to elevated blood sugar levels, and therefore you have excess sugar in your blood stream, which the candida feeds on. So eating lots of chocolate was the worst thing I could have done.

"I have tried many different plans and special diets, but they don't work for me because they don't address diabetes and candida together. Fortunately, I'm studying nutrition, so I'm learning more all the time. And I have to take special care around the time of my period, when the hormonal fluctuation affects the blood sugar levels.

"Colonic irrigation has helped me massively because that clears the candida out of the colon. I feel unbelievably great afterwards, and the candida really settles down, until I get an elevated blood sugar level, or eat something I shouldn't, and then it comes back. I've been taking specialist vitamins and minerals, but there are other things I'd like to try, such as homeopathy.

"My advice to anybody with candida would be to address the diet first. The most important thing is to cut sugar out of the diet in every form, including fruit unfortunately. See a professional who knows which vitamins and minerals would be suitable for you, because everyone will have different requirements."

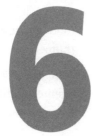

Possible long-term and more serious changes

The menopause is generally thought to bring with it three different types of issues:

- Changes that occur prior to, and around the menopause, such as the ones already mentioned in chapters 4 and 5.

- The intermediate changes, which tend to occur later on in the menopausal process – often after your periods have stopped. These are quite likely to be associated with sagging and dropping, as the muscles and ligaments lose strength and elasticity. Prolapse (sinking down) of the womb or bladder can sometimes occur, although of course this can happen when you are much younger too. And vaginal changes may be more noticeable at this stage as your vaginal tissue becomes thinner.

- Then there are potential long-term concerns that may not manifest until many years afterwards, such as osteoporosis or heart disease.

Here we consider some of these issues. Please bear in mind that you may never experience any of them. It's useful to be informed though, so that you can decide how to deal with them should they arise.

INTERMEDIATE CHANGES

The following are usually associated with the more intermediate changes that can occur during the menopause process.

Hysterectomy

A hysterectomy is an operation to remove the womb. It is done because there is a problem with the womb and only after eliminating other ways to deal with the situation. The need for a hysterectomy is not necessarily a result of menopausal changes, although these can be a factor. The main reasons why a hysterectomy may be recommended are:

Your womb may have prolapsed

That is, the muscles holding it in place have become so weak that your womb drops into your vagina – this tends to occur later on, after your periods have stopped. A hysterectomy is not always recommended – it depends how severe the prolapse is and what else can be done.

You may bleed excessively

Very heavy bleeding at periods (menorrhagia) may occur for a range of reasons. One of these is growths in the muscle of the womb (fibroids). Sometimes a hysterectomy may be recommended if you have fibroids, but this is not the main course of treatment for these unless they are very large. Fibroids are more common in women before reaching the menopause. Some cancers also cause excessive bleeding.

Years ago, you may have expected to have a hysterectomy if you bled excessively, but there are many other ways to deal with this now. So avoid being too alarmed if you have the occasional heavy bleed. It is quite natural for this to happen sometimes as part of the menopause process. Just check how often it occurs, how much blood you are losing, and the colour and texture of it. Talk to the doctor if you have any concerns at all.

You might have endometriosis

There are many ways to deal with this, but sometimes a hysterectomy may be recommended. Endometriosis is when cells from the lining of your womb travel to other parts of your body, for example your rectum and bowel. Each month these cells thicken and bleed, but they can't leave your body in the same way that blood from your womb does, because of where they are. So they remain trapped wherever they are situated – and this can be very painful.

Or it is possible …

You may have cancer of some of the reproductive organs.

If you have a hysterectomy, your womb will be removed. Sometimes, it may be recommended that your ovaries are removed at the same time.

❝ When I was about 40 my periods became incredibly heavy. I was found to be anaemic and was given iron tablets, but the periods continued to get heavier and finally it was discovered that I had fibroids. Apparently one was getting really big and starting to press on my bladder.

I was fitted with a Mirena⁺ coil to lessen the bleeding, but my periods were so heavy that they washed it out — several times. I was losing so much blood and my iron level became so low that I had a blood transfusion, and I was told that I'd need a hysterectomy, which I had when I was 49. I was then put on HRT straightaway, and I was absolutely fine. Having the hysterectomy was the best thing ever. It just sorted things out. Especially for me, because I never wanted children, and my periods had given me a lot of bloody pain and anguish for a very long time. **❞**
Judy, 54

⁺ The contraceptive Mirena coil is fitted inside the womb, where it gradually releases progestogen – a manufactured hormone that has the same effect as progesterone in the body. It makes periods lighter by making the womb lining thin.

If your ovaries are removed

You will go through the menopause soon afterwards because the removal of your ovaries means that your main source of oestrogen is removed too. Therefore this will trigger the menopause.

If your ovaries are not removed

They still produce an egg, but you won't have a period. The egg just dissolves in the pelvis.

You will still go through your usual cycle, as this is controlled by hormones from your ovaries mainly. So if you were prone to pre-menstrual symptoms before your hysterectomy, you will probably continue to get them afterwards.

Generally you will go through the menopause at your natural time, as your ovaries will still be producing oestrogen. But sometimes your oestrogen levels can be affected by having your womb removed. So this could mean that you go through the menopause earlier than you would have expected to, had you not had a hysterectomy. Remember that since everything is connected, one thing affects another.

HRT is often recommended in order to redress the balance, and to help you through potential sudden and uncomfortable menopausal changes that you might experience. Also, if you have had your ovaries removed and you are in, say, your 40s, it may be recommended that you take HRT as the lack of oestrogen for a prolonged period may increase your risk of developing osteoporosis or heart disease. For more on HRT, see page 139.

ff In my mid 30s I started to get horrendous pains with periods, even in my back, and terrible blood loss. It gradually got worse and worse, and I started getting anaemic. I was given a D and C*, and then two weeks later I went on holiday to Florida for a fortnight. I was due to start a period and had terrible backache one day, and then started to bleed really heavily. I took medication which helped the pain but it didn't stop the bleeding. When I got home I was told I had endometriosis, which meant nothing to me, and that my womb was twice the size it should be because of the thickened lining, and odd shape. I was offered a hysterectomy and within a fortnight it was done. I was 39. It wasn't a full hysterectomy because my ovaries weren't removed. I remember the consultant coming into the room and saying to me, 'We'll leave your ovaries in to keep you young and beautiful.' I think that's probably why my menopause has been OK. It took me about six months to start to feel any benefit, and then after another six months I realised it was the best thing I'd ever had. ™™
Trish, 54

*D and C stands for 'dilatation and curettage'. This means that the opening of the neck of the womb is stretched very slightly (dilatation) to allow an instrument through, and the lining is scraped out (curettage) in order to check it under a microscope. This is a short operation that is done under general anaesthetic but it's rarely done now. It has been replaced by telescopes inserted into the cervix – and this is frequently done under local anaesthetic.

Bladder issues

Oestrogen helps your muscles to keep strong and elastic, so it is hardly surprising that as the level of oestrogen diminishes, some of the strength and elasticity in your muscles and ligaments may lessen. In other words, things begin to sag. Added to this, some bodily tissue becomes thinner and drier, for example, the walls of your vagina, and tissue around the whole genital area. All this can lead to trouble with your bladder. Also, the muscles of the pelvic floor which support all your pelvic organs, including your womb, bladder and rectum, lose some of their elasticity, and this can mean that:

- You might not be able to control your bladder and find that you leak urine a little, especially when you sneeze, cough, laugh, lift things and run or jump.

- Things sag to the point of prolapse, so that your womb or bladder sinks down into your vagina, which is of course uncomfortable and needs sorting out.

- You are more prone to bladder and urine infections.

❝ I've got a bladder problem now. It got so bad that I went to see a urinary specialist and I had to see the nurse every few weeks. She gave me loads of exercises to do which helped. I can go for ages without wanting to wee — maybe a couple of hours, but then all of a sudden I think 'I need the toilet', and before I get there, I've started to wet myself. I just can't hold it. It's really frustrating.
Trish, 54 **❞**

It's important to realise that the main cause of problems with the bladder is to do with pelvic floor damage caused by childbirth. Menopause can exacerbate that, but it is not the main cause. Therefore, issues with your bladder can occur at any time, but they tend to be more common around the time of the menopause.

What you can do to help yourself

● Wear absorbent pads to help make leaks less embarrassing.

● Pelvic floor exercises. These are sometimes called Kegel exercises, named after the obstetrician who developed them.

● Bouncing (as mentioned on page 69) is a great way of remembering to do your pelvic floor exercises too. If anything is likely to 'escape', it will want to do so while you bounce – so that'll remind you to do them. *If you have a prolapse it may not be advisable to bounce, so please check with your doctor first.*

Urine infections

Urine infections, which are sometimes referred to as cystitis, can cause real discomfort. The discomfort you experience may well be a sign of infection, but it could just be due to the thinning of the tissues around the bladder, so it's wise to seek medical help so that you get a correct diagnosis.

You might feel that you need to go to the toilet repeatedly, and it may be painful and stinging when you do. Your urine may smell or look cloudy. You might get backache around your kidneys. Urine infections tend to be more common during menopause as the skin around the bladder becomes drier and thinner, and there are fewer bacteria to fight off infection in that area due to the change in vaginal secretions because of the drop in oestrogen. Keep a watch for urine infections. They need treating as soon as possible.

Pelvic floor exercises

The pelvic floor is the sheet of muscles that provides a floor for the organs inside your pelvis and it controls the openings to them. These organs are your womb and vagina, your bladder and urethra, your back passage and anus. Exercising the pelvic floor muscles strengthens them.

Basically, the idea is to squeeze these muscles in the same way that you might do to prevent yourself from urinating. And then release them. There are different recommendations about how many times you should do this and for how long you should hold, but the main message is: frequently, because they are muscles and therefore respond to regular exercise. The important thing is to avoid holding your breath or tightening your buttocks when you do them.

You can do the exercises quickly: squeeze for a second, hold for a second, relax for a second. This helps your pelvic floor to cope with sudden pressure such as when you sneeze or cough. Do it about 10 times in one go, several times a day.

Or do the exercises slowly which helps to really strengthen the muscles: squeezing them to a count of 10, holding for 10 and then letting go. Do 10 of these in one go if you can, several times a day.

Medical warning: it may not be appropriate to do these exercises if you have a urinary infection, so please check with your doctor first.

What you can do to help yourself

- Drink lots of water to keep your system flushed out.

- Avoid caffeine drinks and alcohol (although someone I knew with a urine infection swore that having a couple of vodkas helped).

- Drinking cranberry juice can help.

- Exercise as usual to keep everything working as well as it can.

- Avoid using soap or deodorant around your genitals. If you wear panty liners, wear ones that are unscented.

- Wear cotton underwear so that the genital area can 'breathe'.

- Avoid wearing trousers, tights or underwear that are too tight.

- Wipe from front to back when you go to toilet to avoid transferring bacteria.

- Urinate after sex to flush bacteria away.

LONG-TERM CONCERNS

The following section deals with some of the potential long-term concerns. These may not manifest themselves until many years afterwards. Of course they can occur earlier for some women.

Heart disease

It makes sense that as hormones affect so much of your body's functioning, they must impact upon the state and functioning of your heart. Heart disease is caused by the narrowing of your blood vessels. The type of heart disease you may encounter depends on which blood vessels are affected.

There are a number of risk factors associated with heart disease, so if these apply to you and you are concerned, you may want to talk to your doctor about them. These are:

- A close family history of heart disease.
- High blood pressure.
- High cholesterol level in your blood.
- Smoking.
- Being overweight.
- A lack of exercise.
- Your age.

There is ongoing research into just how much Hormone Replacement Therapy (HRT) may reduce or increase the risk of heart disease. However, it is generally thought that HRT may help to prevent the risk increasing in women who experience early or premature menopause, because it replaces the oestrogen that their bodies would otherwise lack for many years.

High blood pressure

Though there may be no direct link between menopause and high blood pressure, it is something to be mindful of, especially as you get older. Blood pressure rises with age. You might think of it like this: your blood vessels are a plumbing structure, and as time goes on the pipes get a bit worn. They get less compliant, and therefore the pressure on them is higher. The body has to work harder to pump the blood round and circulate it because the arteries are hardening and therefore you require more pressure to get the blood round the system.

But it can be very alarming to discover that your blood pressure is high when you are in your 40s and early 50s. If your blood pressure is consistently high, you run the risk of having a stroke or a heart attack. And the thing is, you don't necessarily know that it *is* high until a reading is taken. You may be ultra-busy, ultra-stressed and into your menopause as well.

Without being obsessive about it, take the issue of your blood pressure seriously. Keep an eye on it, and do what you can to keep it at a reasonable level.

Cholesterol

Cholesterol is a fat (also known as a lipid) made in your liver. It is carried around your body by proteins, and together these are referred to as lipoproteins. Cholesterol is essential for your general health and well-being and is found in every cell in your body. Very basically, there are two types of cholesterol (or lipoproteins): 'good', and 'bad', according to what job they do:

Good – returns cholesterol in the cells to your liver so that it can be broken down, or so that it can leave your body as waste.

Bad – takes cholesterol from your liver to the cells. If there is too much for the cells to use, there will be a build-up. This may mean that it starts to block your arteries, which could then lead to heart disease.

There can be all sorts of reasons why you may have high cholesterol. Some of these could be:

- It rises naturally with age.
- You may have a family history of high cholesterol levels.

- An unhealthy lifestyle, lacking in exercise and a good diet. Also if you smoke, drink too much alcohol or are overweight. The amount your diet affects your cholesterol level varies from one person to another, but in general your liver is likely to produce more 'bad' cholesterol if your diet is high in saturated fats.

- Some health conditions may trigger high cholesterol levels. Some of these are: an under-active thyroid gland, poorly controlled diabetes, and some liver and kidney diseases.

- Some medications may cause cholesterol levels to rise.

- The menopause, and early menopause.

Recent research shows that the menopause has a significant effect because the drop in oestrogen causes your cholesterol levels to rise. This can be measured via a simple blood test. Treatment is usually via medication and a change in diet and lifestyle.

Many women have found that some complementary therapies, combined with a healthy diet and lifestyle, can help to significantly reduce their blood pressure, and their cholesterol level.

❝ I was horrified to find that my blood pressure was sky high. It really worried me. I phoned my homeopath and she said, 'Oh we can do something with that. I can fit you in and we'll start working with it now.' And it's fine now. I have it checked every couple of months, and if it gets a bit high my homeopath sorts it out. **❞**
Janie, 54

❝ You don't necessarily need medication to clear your arteries. There are other things you can take, such as certain vitamins and minerals. The way they work is a bit like descaling a kettle.
Dee, 48 **❞**

What you can do to help yourself

Take advice from the British Heart Foundation. Most of this is around healthy lifestyle and diet, and they have a great website with masses of useful information.

> **British Heart Foundation:**
> www.bhf.org.uk; Heart helpline 0300 330 3311

Osteoporosis

Osteoporosis means that your bones become thinner and more brittle. The bone tissue deteriorates and becomes more fragile, so that your bones break easily. It is called 'the silent epidemic' because most people don't know they've got it until they fall over and break something, especially a wrist, hip or a bone in their spine.

Oestrogen helps to keep bones strong and healthy, so as the level of oestrogen falls at the menopause, your bones become less dense. Risk factors include:

- If a family member has osteoporosis, especially your mother.
- If you have broken bones before.

- Your age – it occurs as you get older.

- If you go through menopause prematurely (before 45).

- Certain medical conditions, and medications you may be taking such as steroids.

- Drinking too much alcohol and smoking.

- Being underweight.

- Your diet – especially a lack of calcium.

- Lack of weight-bearing exercise.

A common time to develop osteoporosis is when you are in your 60s and 70s, although the seeds are sown much earlier, from adolescence onwards. But at the menopause your bones become more fragile as your oestrogen level drops, and this can happen quite quickly if you don't do something about it.

You need, quite simply, to be aware. For a start, enjoy a healthy lifestyle with a good diet and plenty of exercise. Be aware of the risk factors and if they apply to you, discuss your concerns with your doctor. It may be that he or she recommends that you have a bone scan. However there is not currently a national programme for this, as there is for breast screening, so it is not widely available. A bone scan can give you an indication of what your risk is. Then based on that, you may or may not be advised to have some treatment.

Many people are affected by osteoporosis, and you may wonder why there is not a national programme for bone scanning.

66 While the medical treatments recommended for osteoporosis, for example hormone replacement or another drug such as bisphosphonates, are very effective, they all carry risks. They're small, but they're there. So you have to be careful and not just give them to everybody. Clearly if a bone scan revealed that someone had osteoporosis, we would certainly want to do something about it, and offer treatment. However, if someone has been found to have slightly thin bones in their early 50s it may be best not to start any particular treatment at that stage, because potentially that could mean 20–30 years of a treatment which in itself could have side effects and problems.

So, as a general rule, it's probably better not to scan for osteoporosis until the person is in their 60s, unless there are other strong indicators or risks such as an early menopause or strong family history, because usually it's more appropriate to start the treatment then, and the outcome will be just as good. So it's not always a case of 'the sooner the better'.

Tim Hillard, consultant gynaecologist, chairman of the British Menopause Society 99

What you can do to help yourself

- Any weight-bearing exercise – that is, physical activity where you are supporting the weight of your own body, because this makes the bones stronger. So things like brisk walking, jogging and dancing.

- Eat a good, balanced diet and avoid too much salt, caffeine, fizzy drinks and animal protein – all of which can affect the amount of calcium in your body.

- Avoid smoking, and drinking too much alcohol.

- Contact the National Osteoporosis Society, because they can give you the latest recommendations regarding exercise, diet and lifestyle.

National Osteoporosis Society:
www.nos.org.uk; tel 0845 450 0230

Dementia and Alzheimer's disease

Dementia is an umbrella term used to describe various brain disorders that involve a progressive loss of brain function. The most common form is Alzheimer's disease.

Although people experience dementia differently, symptoms include:

- Mood changes.

- Loss of memory – about all sorts of things, such as what you did earlier that day.

- Communication problems, in that your ability to talk, read or write is affected.

- Difficulties carrying out everyday tasks.

Do they sound familiar? If you are going through, or have been through, spates of forgetfulness and confusion, and are aware that you have done the most bizarre things during the menopause process, you may really worry that you could develop some form of dementia, especially if there is a family history of this. But the mental changes you experience during menopause are usually just because of the menopause. They are not an indicator that you will develop dementia.

But it has been suggested that the lack of oestrogen after menopause may be a contributing factor. Therefore treatment with HRT may be recommended. However, some studies have shown there to be no beneficial effect and that HRT may even increase the risk.

To be honest, we are all at risk of developing dementia, because the risk increases with age and the ageing process generally. But there are lots of things we can do to help guard against this, including stimulating your brain with new and interesting activities.

Alzheimer's Society:
www.alzheimers.org.uk; tel 020 7423 3500

NHS Direct:
www.nhs.uk; tel 0845 4647

Cancer

The risk of most types of cancer increases with age, but menopause itself is not thought to be a specific risk factor. Although women can be affected by cancer at any age, it is more common in women over 50 and who have reached menopause. Oestrogen (and of course other hormones as well) does have an effect, and the most common form of cancer among women in the UK is breast cancer.

Different types of breast cancer develop in different parts of the breast. The risk increases with age, therefore in the UK we have an NHS breast screening programme which entitles all women between the ages of 50–70 to be screened once every three years. However, if there is a risk of breast cancer in your family, you may be offered screening earlier.

Breast cancer is usually medically treated with a combination of chemotherapy, radiotherapy and surgery, and in some cases hormone treatments are offered. Chemotherapy could cause you to go through the menopause, if you have not reached this stage naturally beforehand. You are unlikely to be offered HRT if you have breast cancer as this could exacerbate it.

If you notice any changes in your breasts such as a lump or swelling on your breast or in your armpits – or any unusual pain there, or a change in the skin of your breasts, rashes around your nipple, changes in your nipple shape or discharge from your nipples, see your doctor. Be aware though, that lumps in the breast do not necessarily mean that you have cancer.

66 I developed breast cancer. There was no lump – it was detected purely on a mammogram and it was spread over a wide area. There are different types, but mine was to do with the adrenal glands producing too much oestrogen. In some cases, breast cancer cells can be stimulated by oestrogen. I can't have any soya because it would increase oestrogen in my system. I take the drug tamoxifen to block the production. So now I get menopausal symptoms, because I get hot flushes, mood swings and weight gain.

I had hours of surgery and reconstruction work, and from the start of my diagnosis I was determined to become well again. I thought and felt myself into wellness. I don't let things get me down, and I pay more attention to things that inspire and please me. Now I'm really healthy. I eat organic food, I swim, I run three miles each day, and walk several miles before breakfast — which is usually fresh juice and a cocktail of necessary medication and supplements. And I have just qualified to teach yoga.

Lizzie, 54

”

What you can do to help yourself

Develop and maintain a positive attitude, and keep as healthy a lifestyle and diet as you possibly can.

NHS Direct:
www.nhs.uk; tel 0845 4647

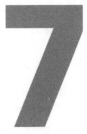

Premature and early menopause

Although definitions of premature and early menopause differ, premature menopause generally refers to women who experience the menopause under the age of 40, whereas early menopause refers to those under the age of 45. Some women are very, very young when they start the menopause – in their 20s or 30s, and even occasionally in their teens.

66 I'd never even thought about the menopause. We'd just started our family – one daughter – but then I just stopped having periods. Eventually the doctor said I'd gone through the menopause. It was a terrible shock.
Jane, 31
99

Women experience premature and early menopause for a variety of reasons:

- It may just happen naturally, without any particular reason.

- It may happen because of a genetic tendency, if, for example, your mother and grandmother had a premature or early menopause. There are also other genetic reasons, such as certain medical conditions that may also run through your family.

- Some treatments for cancer, such as chemotherapy and radiotherapy can affect the ovaries and therefore result in a premature or early menopause.

- Surgery. A hysterectomy that involves the removal of the ovaries as well, triggers an instant menopause. If your womb only was removed, you would expect your ovaries to carry on functioning until you are about 50. Some women who have a hysterectomy find that they go through a slightly earlier menopause than they otherwise would have done because everything is connected and affects everything else. Research shows that about 20% of women who have had their wombs only removed go through menopause earlier because of the surgery.

66 When my friend found out I was taking HRT she said: 'What are you on that for? It's for old people.' I felt so embarrassed — and hurt. It's not my fault that I've gone through the menopause.
Charlotte, 28 **99**

The number of women who experience premature menopause is very small (about 1% of the population in the UK), but is thought to be increasing.

This is because more children and young women survive treatment for cancer now. Some cancer treatments affect the ovaries, which can result in early or premature menopause.

❝Young women find that there's no one else to talk to and they feel alienated. All the literature and books show pictures of women in their late 40s, 50s and 60s. They don't show 20-year-olds. So young women feel very much on their own. They don't want to talk to their friends about it because they feel embarrassed or uncomfortable. They also tend to blame themselves quite often. Things like: 'Have I done something wrong? Should I have eaten something, done something, not had sex with that person?' Of course it's not their fault.

Also, the symptoms are often not as straightforward to recognise as they are in an older person, so some women put a lot of blame on the medical profession. For example, when a young woman goes to the doctor for a problem with her menstrual cycle, the doctor wouldn't usually consider menopause in the first instance. They'd hope that it would be to do with something else, such as a change of diet or over-exercise, or a recent illness that hasn't gone away. But a lot of women say that they feel they've been fobbed off and are not given a referral. It can be months, years even, from the time a woman first goes to see her doctor to getting a correct diagnosis. So that can be a long time of to-ing and fro-ing. Of course, another reason that a diagnosis can take so long is because the woman reckons that she'll be OK the next month, and so doesn't go to the doctor then. But it's a huge emotional rollercoaster, and one of the worst things is having no one in your own peer group to talk to about it.

Amanda Hillard, clinical nurse specialist who runs a menopause clinic **"**

Amanda and other specialists are able to:

- Listen and advise.

- Refer young women to The Daisy Network, a charity dedicated to women who experience premature menopause. Apart from lots of information, this charity enables women to talk to counsellors and to other women who are going through something similar. Their email system, Daisy Mail, enables members to share thoughts and ideas through a central address.

The Daisy Network:
www.daisynetwork.org.uk; daisy@daisynetwork.org.uk

- Put women in contact with other women they can talk to.

- Advise about HRT. Women may choose not to take it, but they should be given all the information. The recommendation from national agencies is that all women who experience early or premature menopause should take HRT until they are 50, because this will be a true replacement of what their bodies would have been producing had they continued to menstruate into, say, their late 40s. Medical professionals say it is vitally important that women who have gone through early and premature menopause consider this, because they have a much higher risk of long-term problems like heart disease and osteoporosis due to the early drop in their oestrogen levels.

66 Sometimes young women who take HRT hear a 'scare story', and so they stop taking it. What they often don't realise is that the risks mentioned are not really relevant to them at their age. They usually relate to women in their late 50s and 60s when the situation is very different.

Tim Hillard, consultant gynaecologist, chairman of the British Menopause Society 99

If you are going through a premature or early menopause it's important to avoid bottling up your thoughts and feelings about it. Seek some help and talk about it. There are many others who are going through the same thing. You are not 'odd' and you are no less a woman just because this has happened to you. A woman's menstrual cycle rules her life – until some time after it has come to an end. If yours has ended sooner than you expected, then you absolutely deserve to take the time to allow this to sink in. It takes time to adjust. And take strength from the fact that right now, many others are adjusting to something similar too.

Caroline

Caroline, *now 45, went through a premature menopause at the age of 39.*

"I was 35 when I had my second child, and 37 when my partner and I split up. When I was 39 I was diagnosed as having been through the menopause.

"I hadn't had a period properly for about three years prior to that diagnosis, though. I'd have them in the winter months, and then go the whole summer without having any at all. And I had horrendous moods. I got very low, and was quick to snap at people. But I thought it was all down to stress. I was having difficulty coping with the breakdown of my relationship, and my eldest child was an out-of-control teenager. Now, looking back, I think it was also linked to the hormonal imbalance going on in my body. But of course I wasn't aware of that at the time.

"When my partner left I went into a breakdown and didn't eat. My 14-year-old was drinking and really difficult to deal with. Everything seemed to happen at once. Not eating was just my way of coping. So I had all these things going on together, and eventually I thought I better get checked out, so I went to the doctor and a blood test showed that I was perimenopausal. Soon after that that my periods stopped completely.

"When this was diagnosed I was so upset and angry. I was spoken to about HRT and given a leaflet to read about it, but I thought, 'I don't need HRT. That's for old people, and I'm a young woman.' I felt young, and the menopause – well, I would never have expected to think about that until I was in my 50s. But I did start taking Ymea, which is a food supplement made from plant extracts, to aid the menopause.

"The way I dealt with everything is that I gave myself a hard time. I blamed myself. I gave myself a hard time because I thought that maybe this had happened because I'd stopped eating and lost so much weight. I know periods can stop with stress and massive weight loss, so I blamed myself for that. And I continued not to eat. I carried on being angry for a very long time.

"I do think an early menopause probably had quite a lot to do with the breakdown of my relationship, because of the mood swings I had. Some of them must have been attributable to hormonal changes, but I didn't know that at the time.

"Having to go to work was a mixed blessing really. In many ways it was light relief compared to everything else I had to deal with. But there was a lot of discontent among my colleagues, and I know they had the impression that I was a moody, miserable bitch. Which I was. But fair play to me, at least I survived.

"My advice to anyone going through an early menopause is to keep your head down, grit your teeth and just get on with it, because it does get better. It honestly does get better."

part three

Choosing a treatment

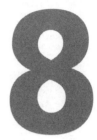

Treatments available

Many women just go through their menopause – and that's it. They appear to experience little real discomfort, and if they do they just accept it and get on with their lives. They don't seek any help, and a few years later say they never really noticed it.

On the other hand, many women are acutely aware of the changes taking place. They are uncomfortable and fed up with the way they feel, and they want some help and support.

❝My impression is that there are essentially two schools of thought about how to deal with menopause. One is medical. Women come to doctors and nurses with symptoms or problems, and a solution is recommended. For that, as professionals, we tend to look at what evidence we have, and the evidence is largely in favour of using hormones, because in the majority of cases, they work very well.

The other school of thought is a leave alone and let nature take its course approach, which says that the menopause is a natural event and you don't need hormones to manage it. Both can be right — there's no right or wrong in this.

The trouble with all the information available over the internet, and in books and magazines, is that they tend to favour one approach or the other, so it's quite hard to get a balance, and a balanced approach is usually best.

Tim Hillard, consultant gynaecologist, chairman of the British Menopause Society

"

If you seek help through the medical route, this usually means taking a course of HRT or some other form of medication. There is also a range of complementary therapies which many women find very helpful, although these may not be scientifically proven. Some women report that they have benefited from other less well-known or esoteric therapies. And there is a huge range of products and supplements on sale which you can buy according to what you fancy, and what is likely to benefit you most at the time.

It's never too late, or too soon, to find out about different treatments and therapies, and how they may be able to help you. This may seem like a daunting task, but you don't need to know *everything*. Just see what appeals to you, and find out something about it. It's important to do some research, otherwise you won't know what to expect.

There's no point in going to a reflexologist if you hate having your feet touched, or having acupuncture if your fear of needles is so great that it triggers an anxiety attack.

It's perhaps important to mention that there is a school of thought that says that if you have or do something that you think will make you better, it probably will because you are expecting it to - regardless of its healing properties. So if you ate a Magic Toffee that you believed was able to alleviate every discomfort you could experience that day, you would probably feel fine all day. But then, you might have felt fine all day anyway, whether you'd eaten the toffee or not. You'd never know really. (Of course, there may have been no magical properties to the toffee at all, but you believed there were.) This is what's known as the placebo effect.

So where do you start? It's important to be informed about the choices available, and then you can decide what might be best for you. However there is so much information out there that it can be utterly baffling.

One important treatment to have some knowledge of is HRT, because medically this is the treatment of choice for menopause-related issues. Some women know nothing about, and have no wish to know anything about, HRT. They are happy to take it because it makes them feel better. They are happy to take the advice of medical professionals, who are the experts. And of course that's true - medical professionals *are* experts, and they have vast amounts of knowledge about what works, based on clinical trials and research and evidence.

But many women have been helped by using other therapies and treatments, and it's important to be informed so that you can make choices - if you want to.

The key to a smooth menopause seems to be balance. Every medical and complementary health practitioner that I spoke to while researching this book stressed the importance of that. And so did many of the women who told me their own stories.

It's about taking a balanced approach, and being sensible. It's about being informed and aware of what is happening to you, and the choices available. Yet at the same time, it is true that some women are happy to take what is offered to them without question – and that's fine. It has to be whatever works for you as an individual, and what you feel most comfortable with.

So in this next section, we'll consider HRT first. After that, we'll look at a range of complementary therapies that women have found to be beneficial during the menopause. This will help you to make an informed decision about what might be best for you.

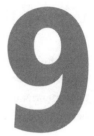

Hormone Replacement Therapy (HRT)

If you go to the doctor because you are experiencing discomfort around your menopause, you may be offered HRT.

❝ When I moved house I was 51. I went to register with the doctor, and when they saw my age they said, 'You'll be wanting to see the HRT nurse, I expect.' And I said 'No, thank you.' I subsequently discovered that it was misleading because she's not the 'HRT nurse'. She advises people about the menopause. ❞

Sally, 58

WHAT IS HRT?

Hormone replacement therapy (HRT) does just what it says. It replaces the levels of hormones that reduce naturally throughout the menopause process. The main hormones involved are oestrogen and progesterone, as these are the ones that decline.

Basically, HRT is used to treat and relieve some of the changes that can occur at the menopause, and many women find that it is very helpful. Research has shown that it may also prevent osteoporosis, and possibly some forms of dementia. HRT is also often recommended when the menopause happens suddenly, for example as a result of having the ovaries removed, or in the cases of early or premature menopause. This is because the ensuing sudden loss of oestrogen could cause problems later on. More of this later.

WHAT DO YOU TAKE?

Most women who use HRT will take oestrogen, as this is the hormone that is so important for women, as well as progesterone, to stop the lining of the womb growing too much. (Remember, progesterone keeps oestrogen in control and regulates what it does.) However, if you have had a hysterectomy and your womb has been removed, you do not need progesterone. Sometimes, you might take testosterone as well, especially if your ovaries have been removed. (One of the places that produces testosterone in women is the ovaries.)

The other female sex hormones, FSH and LH, are not generally thought to cause any specific changes throughout the menopause process. Their levels just get higher to try to encourage the ovaries to work again. High levels of FSH and LH are just regarded as markers; that is, they indicate that your oestrogen level is low.

All hormones are chemicals

It's important to understand that all hormones are chemical by definition. They are the body's chemical messengers. The hormones used in HRT are compounds that are manufactured in a laboratory, but are made from naturally occurring substances, in the same way that something like, say, evening primrose oil is manufactured by a process in order to turn it into a tablet. Most of the oestrogens are derived from plant extracts. One type is derived from horse urine, and is the most widely available in the world, but it is being used less frequently.

The progesterone that circulates in your body is very different from the natural progesterone that is available to buy in gels or creams. The progesterone that is prescribed for medical purposes such as HRT is a manufactured hormone, which is either the same as, or similar to, the progesterone in your body. It is a drug which needs a licence and has undergone rigorous trials.

So the two are quite different, and there is a lot of confusion about this. Natural progesterone cream or gel is much weaker. Many women have benefited from taking it and have found that it has helped to relieve hot flushes, but it is not the same as medical progesterone, and so shouldn't be confused with it or compared to it.

HOW DO YOU TAKE IT?

Oestrogen is most commonly taken in tablet form or a patch. It can also be taken as a gel or you may be given an implant. If it's taken specifically to help with vaginal or urinary symptoms, it can be taken as a cream, vaginal tablet or pessary. Progesterone is taken in tablet form or patch, vaginal gel or through the fitting of a Mirena contraceptive coil, which slowly releases progesterone into the body. If testosterone is recommended it is either taken in the form of a patch, or as a pellet inserted just under the skin.

How frequently you take your tablets, creams, gels or patches depends on what it is and the dosage you require. It could be daily or weekly, or twice-weekly – and there are several routes.

HRT is not something you can prescribe for yourself. Of course, you choose whether you want to use it or not, but each woman's needs are different, and what is given and for how long has to be carefully balanced with your own particular needs at any given stage in your menopause – so your treatment can change and be adjusted accordingly.

Avoid being confused by terminology you might read such as *sequential therapy*, or *cyclical therapy*, or *sequential combined therapy*, or *continuous combined therapy*. It's far better to have a chat with your doctor or specialist nurse so that you can be clear about what is being recommended for you and why.

" The thing about hormones is that you cannot generalise. No two women are the same. What suits one doesn't always suit the next. Some women are what I call 'oestrogen positive '. Their bodies like oestrogen. It makes them feel better. They feel good when they're pregnant, good when they're on the pill, they feel good generally. Then they go through the menopause and they feel lousy and you give them the hormone replacement and they feel well again. Other women don't seem to be so happy with oestrogen and they often don't feel well during pregnancy and when it comes to menopause, they actually feel a bit better as their oestrogen decreases.

The other hormone which is important is progesterone. This has good effects and bad effects. Often in terms of hormone replacement it's seen as the bad guy because it often causes more side effects. But there are some women whose bodies like progesterone.

Menopause is an event but it's only one event in terms of hormonal life span. It starts with puberty, goes through all the reproduction cycles, and for many this includes the whole process of having children, including being ante-natal, post-natal, breast feeding and so on, and then into the menopause. So the menopause is just a phase in a lifelong hormonal cycle, and if you talk to people closely enough you can often pick up a trend by talking to them about how they were during their previous 20 or 30 years.

Tim Hillard, consultant gynaecologist, chairman of the British Menopause Society

"

You cannot possibly be expected to know all about HRT. It's complicated, and though it's useful to be informed, there are all sorts of things to consider when it's prescribed, because interfering with your hormonal system is a big thing.

When you talk to your doctor about this, the following will be discussed and consideration is given to:

- Your age.

- The changes you are experiencing.

- Other possible reasons for some of these changes – for example, your thyroid gland may not be working as well as it used to.

- What stage of your menopause you are at.

- How any treatment is likely to interact with other medications you may be taking.

From there you will be prescribed a specific treatment, at a particular dosage. Then it needs to be monitored carefully, to check that you are absorbing the hormones properly and that it is working well for you. It is recommended that you stick with it for at least three to six months in order to get the full benefit, but it's generally not recommended to stay on HRT for more than a few years.

This way, you'll be able to tell whether or not you still need it, and this should be reviewed regularly with your doctor. Some women may need to stay on HRT for longer though. And avoid taking yourself off HRT suddenly. This needs to be done properly, under supervision, otherwise you may experience unnecessary discomfort.

Your doctor or specialist nurse should be able to tell you what you need to know about HRT and answer any questions that you have relating to its suitability for you. Beware of doing too much detailed research yourself. – there is so much information available and not all of it is useful.

Menopause Matters:
This website is recommended by specialists. It is written by doctors and nurses and gives detailed, current information: www.menopausematters.co.uk

If you do not feel that your questions are answered satisfactorily, keep on asking until you are satisfied. You have a right to know – it's your body and your life, after all.

If you have a particularly early or premature menopause, the recommendation for using HRT may be different. You may be advised to take HRT for several years in order to replace hormones that would naturally have been produced by your body had you not reached your menopause early.

❝ There is a difference between a 50-year-old woman who goes through the menopause and a 30-year-old. There is very clear evidence that early menopause increases the risk of long-term problems such as osteoporosis and heart disease, and possibly dementia as well. The reason for this is that if a woman undergoes her menopause at, say, 30, then she will have 20 years without oestrogen before she is 50, and if this is not treated then she may run into these problems relatively early.

It is strongly recommended by the vast majority of experts that a woman who undergoes menopause early should be given HRT up to the age of 50 as a true replacement hormone – for example, in the same way that you would use thyroxin for thyroid replacement. This is different from prescribing HRT to women beyond the age of 50 where it's primarily being used to treat the symptoms.

Tim Hillard, consultant gynaecologist, chairman of the British Menopause Society ❞

THE BENEFITS OF TAKING HRT

Many women have found that HRT has helped to relieve the following:

- Hot flushes and night sweats.

- Mood swings.

- Insomnia.

- Aches and pains.

- Vaginal dryness and discomfort.

- Urinary infections.

Research has also shown that HRT can help to prevent the onset of osteoporosis (weak and brittle bones). It is thought that it may also help to prevent certain cancers, heart disease and possibly dementia including Alzheimer's disease.

> **❝** I started having really heavy periods. I'd bleed for a month at a time, then stop for a week, and then it would start again. It was making me so ill. My hot flushes were every 10 minutes I couldn't sleep and my blood pressure was far too low. So I was put on HRT.
>
> It's been fantastic. Everything went back to normal. I'm on the very lowest dose – it's literally an underlying dose. So my periods are as they were before, and the hot flushes are almost non-existent. And I can sleep at night. Being on HRT has really changed my life for the better. I

didn't really have any side-effects, except for the fact that I was a bit nauseous and my breasts were quite tender at first — but then within two months I was fine.

Joan, 52

"

THE RISKS OF TAKING HRT

It is thought that the following risks of taking HRT are small, but they are risks none the less:

- There is a slight increase in the risk of certain cancers, particularly of the breast, womb, and possibly the ovaries.
- Blood clots, such as deep vein thrombosis.
- Some heart disease.
- Stroke.

Research shows that risks develop or increase depending on the type of HRT you take and for how long. So this is another reason why it is good to be informed and to talk to your doctor about this.

Generally, HRT is predominantly safe, but the benefits, risks and side effects of it are under constant scrutiny and research is ongoing. You might like to look at the current research on www. menopausematters.co.uk which gives details of relevant studies and statistics.

It is unlikely that you will be prescribed HRT if:

- You are pregnant or breastfeeding.

- You have blood-clotting conditions such as some types of heart disease, for example, angina or a heart attack, or blood clots in your legs or lungs.

- You have some types of cancers – that is, those that are hormone-dependent such as cancer of the breast or womb.

- You have severe liver disease.

- You have vaginal bleeding which is undiagnosed.

- You have an undiagnosed lump in your breast.

POSSIBLE SIDE-EFFECTS OF TAKING HRT

You may experience side-effects, especially in the first two to three months of taking HRT. Without going into great detail, the side-effects you might experience are related to the particular hormones you take. So if after a couple of months you still experience unpleasant or uncomfortable side-effects, go back to your doctor.

> ❝ I didn't take any HRT when I had the hysterectomy, but I did when I started getting hot flushes. It changed my personality – I was like two different people. So I was taken off that after about two months and put on another one, but I didn't feel that it was making any difference at all. I took that one for about three months and that was it. I didn't think I needed it really,

and my experience of it was not good. I reckon I've been fine without it.

Trish, 54

99

The following are common side-effects, but you might have others too:

- Feeling sick and digestive problems.

- Heavy or irregular bleeding if you are still having periods anyway, and possibly some light bleeding if your periods had already stopped.

- Fluid retention and bloating. The fluid retention can occur in different parts of your body such as your face, ankles, legs, breasts and around your waist.

- You may get worse pre-menstrual symptoms than you are used to, or you may get fewer.

- Cramp, especially in your legs.

- Headaches or migraines.

- Aches and pains.

- Mood swings.

- Changes in your skin, such as itching, or developing spots.

As you read this list you might think, 'But those are the things I wanted to relieve. I didn't want them as side-effects.' Well, just remember that everyone is different. If you have masses of hot flushes and have never had a headache in your life, you may be delighted to experience headaches for a few weeks in order to find something that makes the hot flushes subside. The idea is that everything should settle eventually and you will start to feel good again.

> 66 After about four years I thought I probably didn't need HRT any more, so I stopped taking it. But my moods really changed for the worse. So I went back on it, and stuck with it for a while. Then a year ago I decided to wean myself off, and it was better this time. About two or three months afterwards, though, I started to get hot flushes. Sometimes I'd get two or three a day, and other days none at all.
>
> Judy, 54 99

Sally

Sally, *58, had six years of hot flushes and night sweats which affected her entire lifestyle. Acupuncture helped her, and her flushes diminished considerably but are still around.*

"It started at 52. I was having 10-minute hot flushes every 20 minutes throughout every day and night. It was awful. It lasted for about 18 months. At night my whole body was hot. I wasn't drenched with sweat, but I'd be desperate for cool air. I'd want to run out of the door into a cold night, flapping at my body to help the air circulate. I've been through a number of years of not being able to wear make-up because it just slides off my face. It's really annoying. I'd go everywhere looking pale and interesting - well, I'd start off that way and within five minutes I'd look as if I'd just been pulled out of a cauldron.

"I did consider HRT because I was so desperate, but I just don't feel they know enough about it. Having said that,

I have a number of friends who take it and they look fantastic. They don't have make-up slithering down their necks, they're calm, and they can sleep at night. But I decided that I would rather do something that I felt was more natural. I had acupuncture and it was very helpful, even though it emptied my wallet. It was based on removing the dampness from my body. I only did it for about six months because I just couldn't afford it. When I stopped, although the hot flushes came back, they were far less frequent.

"I think that if I was still in the job I had had before, I wouldn't be able to do it. I was constantly having to make decisions, sit through meetings, and deal with people talking at me all the time. It's embarrassing when you're bright red in the face and literally running with sweat. You know that you look awful, and you know that people are noticing and thinking, 'Oh she's at that age.' It's no good saying, 'Sorry I'm having a hot flush.' People don't want to have it pointed out to them. They know you are, but they don't know what to say if you draw attention to it. Women of a similar age or who are going through it are fine though. I work from home now, and I'm so grateful for that, because when it got too much I could just walk away from my computer and run my wrists under a cold tap, or go and change my clothes.

"I'm aware that I don't seem to be able to remember things as well as I should. I can watch a film, thoroughly enjoy it and then afterwards have no idea what it was about. And the same with reading a book. Sometimes I don't even get to the end of the page.

"The menopause is a huge thing. I've never felt saddened by it as some women have, and it puts a lot of things in a different light. I feel that as one door closes another opens. And I suppose I've saved a lot of money on tampons. It's rather nice being able to avoid virtually a whole aisle of the supermarket. It reduces shopping time."

Niki

Niki, 56, has been determined to have as smooth a menopause as possible, and has found complementary therapies to suit her.

"When I was about 49 I started to have lots of mood swings. I was snappy and irritable. My periods were always regular – more or less every 28 days, but when I was about 50 we were away on holiday and I missed one. So I thought I was pregnant, because I had all the signs - but I wasn't. It was quite odd. When I got to about 51 I still carried on having normal periods and then I'd miss one again. And then all of a sudden at about 52 – they just stopped.

"Sometimes it's difficult to know what's caused by the menopause and what's caused by stress, because of the things you experience at that time of your life. It's a difficult time for a woman because it's quite hard when the children flee the nest, and I think you can get very emotional. According to my husband, I could be quite tricky to live with. Sometimes I'd be absolutely fine, and everything was great, and then all of a sudden I'd be a snappy crocodile.

"That's when I thought I ought to start looking into doing something about it. I was determined that the menopause wasn't going to affect me badly. I decided to cope with the menopause myself as it evolves, and try and relieve any problems by natural methods. It hasn't been too bad at all. I'm fortunate in that I don't have hot flushes all the time, like some women do. It does help talking to friends about it. Then you know you're not on your own.

"In the last year-and-a-half I've noticed lots of joint aches in my shoulders and elbows and slightly into my wrists. I think some of this is tension; I sometimes notice aches in my knees too. That's why I think it's important to exercise. I've found walking and tai chi very helpful.

"I think the menopause can exacerbate anxiety. Someone suggested I see a hypnotherapist and it really helped. Once you start on all this, it gets you thinking, and it opens your mind to other ideas and other areas. I've tried lots of different things – reflexology for example, which was excellent. You have to make a decision about what you're going to stick with, and what's working for you. I take a herbal product now, which is a mixture of various herbs, and I find it works very well for me. I still get hot flushes but they're nothing like as intense as they were.

"There's no need to be frightened or worried about the menopause because we all go through it, although it must be devastating to go through it when you are very young. I think that for a lot of women it can be a tricky time, because you feel that you're coming to the end of your youth and your attractiveness. Suddenly you think, 'Oh God, I'm not sexy any more.' But then you accept it in a different way. It can give you a nice, comfortable feeling with yourself eventually. For example, I am much more relaxed in myself, and feel that I can face things straight-on now. A lot of that has come through learning about what's happening to me and exploring alternative ways of managing it. It's been a valuable time."

10

Complementary therapies

The majority of complementary therapies take a holistic approach and work to bring the body into balance on every level. Some treatments include an element of relaxation, although this can also be a sort of by-product of the treatment itself. In other words you may feel blissfully relaxed after being treated for, say, a bladder problem or a digestive issue, or a hot flush.

66 The menopause can often be a challenging time for women physically, psychologically and emotionally. As a holistic therapist I know that there are many ways in which we can help our bodies overcome a lot of these difficulties. Lots of symptoms can be relieved, reduced and even prevented by making sometimes subtle changes to our lifestyles, such as diet, exercise and relaxation. And we need to be able to talk about how we feel.

Jean Nurse, complementary health practitioner 99

Sometimes women ask their doctors whether or not they should try certain complementary therapies, and whether or not they work. But unless that therapy has been proven by masses of clinical research, it may not be recommended as the treatment of choice by medical health professionals. And most complementary therapies have not been scientifically proven. A minute percentage of the national research budget gets spent on any form of complementary medicine, so funding for this is not widely available.

For a fact sheet on current medical thinking about some complementary therapies and their effectiveness at the menopause, see the British Menopause Society's website: www.thebms.org.uk or Menopause Matters: www.menopausematters.co.uk

The following selection of therapies has helped many women through the menopause. Some have been used instead of, or alongside, medical treatment. Of course, there are many therapies available other than those mentioned here – they could fill another book. The following are the ones that many women I spoke to had used. Many complementary therapies take a holistic approach, and often the first consultation can be fairly lengthy. One woman said, 'It can be so reassuring to feel that someone is working **with** your idiosyncrasies, instead of trying to straighten them out.'

If you wish to use a complementary therapy, and are taking medication of some kind, please check with your practitioner that it is safe for you to do both.

Making the most of complementary treatments

If you are considering a complementary treatment, find out the main governing body (or bodies) for that therapy. They will give you good, up-to-date information, plus a list of practitioners that are properly trained. It is useful to have a conversation with a practitioner so that they can answer your questions directly. If you think you would like some treatment with them, ask them about their qualifications, if they've treated something similar before, how long treatment is likely to take and how many appointments you will need, and how much they charge. Alternative and complementary treatment can be very expensive, and sometimes people find that they just can't do it financially if they need to keep going back.

If you don't have one already, check out some private medical insurance plans. Some plans will pay a fair percentage of the complementary practitioner's fee for a relatively small contribution from you each month. But make sure that the treatment you choose is covered by the plan you take out.

When you have chosen a practitioner, tell them everything they need to know. Avoid hiding anything from them. A good practitioner will give you an honest opinion as to whether or not their therapy is likely to help you. There are certain conditions where it may actually be dangerous to receive treatment in a particular therapy. Your therapist cannot advise you if you haven't told them about it.

If you are looking to buy supplements and herbal remedies, and want advice as to what might be best for you, speak to a practitioner such as a herbalist or a nutritionist. There are so many products available to buy, and they are not cheap. The main thing is to find what works for you.

MEDICAL HERBALISM

For many years women have maintained that herbs have helped them during the menopause, and they are readily available to buy over the internet, at health food shops and supermarkets. Individual herbal remedies such as black cohosh and red clover have all been researched, tried, tested and shown to be effective. But to get the best out of herbal medicines it will help to see a qualified practitioner. That way, you'll be sure to get the right remedy for you as an individual. Another thing to be aware of is that herbs are very powerful. They can interact with all sorts of things, such as with foods and with conventional medication. So if you are taking conventional medication, it is really important to seek good advice. A properly trained herbalist will have completed a three- or four-year training and will be up-to-date with continuing professional development. So they will know exactly what you can and can't mix.

Because so many women and practitioners have found that herbal medicine has successfully treated menopausal symptoms, a study into this was recently undertaken by the National Institute of Medical Herbalists (NIMH) in collaboration with the University of Central Lancashire and the United Bristol Healthcare Trust. 'Changing with herbs – treatment of menopause by qualified herbal practitioners' was a randomised control trial, coordinated by Julia Green, who explains how it was carried out.

❝ We worked with a local GP practice and we recruited a sample of 45 women. Some were treated by a herbal practitioner straight away, and some went on a waiting list. We then compared the menopausal symptoms between the two groups, and the women who were treated by herbalists were found to have a significant reduction in their menopausal symptoms. The treatment was particularly successful in reducing hot flushes and night sweats and at increasing sex drive.

A record was kept of the herbs used, and there were several in each prescription. Often these were changed at different phases of the treatment to reflect what each woman needed at the time. So it would be impossible to say that a specific herb would be used to treat a particular symptom, because each treatment was tailored specifically for each individual. In all, over 80 herbs were used in 145 different prescriptions.

After the study, we interviewed the women who took part and asked them what they felt about it and whether or not it had been helpful. Every woman who had treatment said it was helpful.

Julia Green BSc, PhD, FNIMH

"

Medical herbalism, along with many other complementary therapies, takes a holistic approach – in other words, it looks at the person as a whole.

" What you really need to do is to look at everything that's going on in a woman's life. This is vital because each individual is different and there may be important underlying issues. In our study, women came with a range of symptoms, including hot flushes, night sweats, headaches, digestion issues, lack of sex drive, aching joints, and breast tenderness. Some were depressed or anxious. And often women were very tired. So you need to see what else is going on, and what could be contributory factors.

For instance, hot flushes might be exacerbated by diet and stress, and lack of libido could be due to a range of things, such as vaginal changes and discomfort during sex, fatigue — maybe waking up several times a night with night sweats, and feeling low generally.

Julia Green BSc, PhD, FNIMH   **"**

So, typically, if you visit a medical herbalist you can expect a long consultation. You will be listened to, and asked appropriate questions so that he or she can build up a picture of you as a whole. You will be asked about your symptoms, but also about your life in general. So from the discussion, and anything else that may be appropriate (such as taking your blood pressure), the practitioner will come up with a strategy to deal with the symptoms and any underlying issues that could be contributing. This will involve using some herbal remedies, usually given in the form of a tincture, but it will also include explanations and, if appropriate, suggestions for some lifestyle changes.

The women who took part in the study were all interviewed afterwards and asked what changes they had noticed in their symptoms, and also what they felt about the treatment as a whole. All the women said that they really valued being able to talk things through with practitioners who listened to them in a non-judgemental way. Women liked to be able to discuss particular aspects of their lifestyle, such as their diet, and to be given advice in a way that was easy to take. Many said that it was helpful to learn how to do things differently. Women also valued the fact that, where necessary, they were referred to their GP.

The National Institute of Medical Herbalists (NIMH):
www.nimh.org.uk; info@nimh.org.uk; tel 01392 426022

CHINESE HERBAL MEDICINE

Chinese herbal medicine is part of the wider system of Traditional Chinese Medicine (TCM). TCM is one of the world's oldest medical systems. It incorporates acupuncture, therapeutic massage and other techniques. It is a holistic method of treatment that works to balance the functioning of the entire body.

The way that conditions are diagnosed is different from the way that medical practitioners diagnose in the West, because the culture and philosophy of health and medicine is different. So it may help you to bear this in mind when seeking treatment, because it may be a completely different approach from anything you are used to.

Most people around the world use herbs as their traditional medicine, using whatever grows in their own area. So there will be differences between the herbs used in one area of the world and those in another, such as the Amazon rainforest, South Africa, Mexico, the Australian outback, North America, China, India or Europe. But trading has meant that herbs have been brought to Europe from all over the world, and now some are commonly used in both Chinese and European herbal medicine. As with western medical herbalism, many women have found this helpful at menopause.

The Association of Traditional Chinese Medicine (UK):
The main regulatory body for the practice of Chinese herbal medicine in the UK.
www.atcm.co.uk; info@atcm.co.uk; tel 020 8951 3030

Acupuncture

Acupuncture is a holistic therapy, so a treatment is devised specifically for the individual following a careful diagnosis by the practitioner. Traditional Chinese philosophy maintains that a person's overall health depends on the energy known as qi (pronounced 'chi') flowing smoothly through a series of channels (meridians) beneath the skin. All sorts of things can disturb this flow, from emotional and mental issues to physical causes such as nutrition or infections. Fine needles are inserted into these channels to stimulate the body to heal itself and rebalance its energy flow.

No needles

Acupressure is where a therapist places pressure on the body at the same points used in acupuncture. Needles are not used at all.

Often the acupuncture points where the needles are inserted may be nowhere near where you experience your symptoms, but there are about 500 acupuncture points on the body and the acupuncturist will know exactly which to choose.

It's a shame that the needles are called 'needles' because in some ways they are more like firm pieces of thread since they are so very fine. So it's not like having an injection or anything. I spoke to several women who felt that acupuncture had really helped them during menopause. Some had been to acupuncturists who were trained in TCM, and some had been to therapists who practised acupuncture only, or in conjunction with another therapy.

❝ I decided to try acupuncture and TCM. The doctor asked me lots of questions to establish that I was in the menopause. She looked at my tongue for quite a while and took my pulse. Then I was told that I would have acupuncture, but that I would need some herbs which would cost extra but they were an important part of the treatment.

I lay on a couch behind a screen and I was covered with a blanket. And then the doctor inserted these really fine needles into various areas — there were probably about eight or ten that she used. But it didn't hurt at all.

Then I was left on my own. I experienced a throbbing in one of my calves, and I began to panic because it was sore. When I told the doctor, she explained that this was to do with my bladder, and it was good. After a few minutes more, she removed the needles and gave me my herbs which I was told to boil up each day and drink the liquid.

I dutifully prepared them twice a day. They smelt disgusting, and tasted absolutely foul. But I drank the whole lot, and I had a general sense of well-being for months after that. I never got so much as a cold, and my energy level was heaps better.
Shirley, 51 **❞**

> **British Acupuncture Council:**
> www.acupuncture.org.uk; info@acupuncture.org.uk;
> tel 020 8735 0400

AYURVEDA

This is a system of holistic health care that originated in India thousands of years ago. Ayurveda means 'the science of life', and it is concerned with treating disease, preventing ill health and enhancing the quality of life. The basic philosophy is that the universe is composed of five basic elements: air, fire, water, ether (or space) and earth. These elements are thought to be present in all things, and in the human body these are recognised as doshas.

This system of medicine and health care is mentioned here because, like Traditional Chinese Medicine, it originated in a culture outside the Western world and therefore has a very different approach to diagnosing illness. Ayurveda is the traditional medical system of India, where it is used widely. It is fascinating, and has treated many women successfully as they have gone through the menopause.

> **Ayurveda Practitioners' Association:**
> For a comprehensive explanation of Ayurveda, and to find a therapist or practitioner (and there is a difference here, as the association will explain), contact the Ayurvedic Practitioners' Association: www.apa.uk.com; tel 07985 984 146

Homeopathy

Homeopathy works on the principle that 'like cures like'. In other words, a condition can be treated by a substance that would produce similar symptoms in a healthy person. Therefore in order to prescribe an appropriate remedy, the homeopath treats each person as an individual case, looking at every aspect of that person's life – the physical, mental, emotional and spiritual. A remedy that is prescribed for one person may be different from that prescribed for another who has similar symptoms. Remedies are made from plant, mineral, metal and insect sources, and are prescribed in various dilutions and potencies. They stimulate the body to heal itself.

Many women have found that homeopathy has helped them throughout the menopause process, as hormonal imbalances seem to respond well to homeopathic treatment. As with most complementary therapies, you can expect a lengthy, detailed consultation that takes into account all aspects of your life.

❝ The most important thing is that you have to be prepared to talk about exactly what's going on and not hold things back. I need details, and they may need to be graphic. So you have to be open to that. For example, with periods, I may need to know the colour of your flow, how lumpy it is, when it's painful, and so on. And with hot flushes, you need to be able to tell me where in your body they start and exactly how they affect you. Similarly with moods and emotions – it's not enough just to say 'I feel irritable'. I need to know the details – how, when, where.

The more I know, the more I can help. Even if I ask you about something which doesn't seem relevant I can assure you that it will be. It could make all the difference to what I prescribe for you.

One of the great things about homeopathy is that you don't need to come very often, and you can take your remedies away with you, which often includes a back-up. I personally often give a couple of remedies, so that if you're not feeling better after the first one, you can take the other — and then that usually does the trick.

A practising homeopath

99

66 I've been into homeopathy for about 25 years. Because I have moved areas several times, I have had to find a different homeopath each time, and they have all been different in their approach. For example, the first I went to was also a medical doctor. My current homeopath is also a reflexologist, and it is wonderful going to see her because the whole environment is so relaxing.

I'm sure I'm in the menopause. I haven't had a period for a few months and I've been very up and down emotionally. Seeing her has really helped. It's good to be able to talk about everything and she always seems to give me a remedy that settles me. She's also given me something to take should I feel myself getting agitated, which is reassuring.

I'd never just go and buy a remedy — I'd far rather see my homeopath and get the right thing for me. So I tend not to take anything else — no other supplements or anything. I'd always ask her first now, because I know she'll recommend the stuff that will work well for me.
Rachel, 48

"

Alliance of Registered Homeopaths:
www.a-r-h.org; tel 08700 736339

Society of Homeopaths:
www.homeopathy-soh.org; tel 0845 450 6611

Aromatherapy

Aromatherapy involves the use of essential oils extracted from plants. Leaves, roots, flowers, berries, stems and bark are all used, and the oils extracted are very potent and should be used with care. An aromatherapist will carefully choose and blend a number of oils together to enhance their therapeutic effect, depending on what they are to be used for. Then you'll be shown how to use them. They can be inhaled, put in the bath, used in hot or cold compresses, or used in an aromatherapy massage.

The Aromatherapy Council:
www.aromatherapycouncil.co.uk; tel 0870 774 3477

> **❝**I have successfully treated many women for various
> menopausal symptoms, and specific oils are known to be
> particularly useful at this time. For example, geranium is
> great for balancing hormones, clary sage helps with hot
> flushes and night sweats, and ylang ylang regulates hormones
> and increases libido. And then there are several which
> uplift generally and help with emotional issues. It's complex,
> and you do have to be careful, because if someone has a
> medical condition, using some oils could be dangerous.
>
> Jean Nurse, complementary health practitioner **❞**

REFLEXOLOGY

A reflexologist uses the hands to apply pressure to the feet. This can feel like a massage or it may take the form of a very light touch to certain areas. Each part of the foot has reflex points that correspond to different parts of the body. If there are energy blockages in the body for any reason, such as illness or stress, a reflexologist can detect these as tiny deposits and imbalances, and can release them by working on the appropriate parts of the foot.

Many therapists believe that there are such things as 'energy blockages', although these tend to be undefined. Once the blockages are released, the affected area is free to heal itself and return to normal.

Reflexology does not work specifically on acupuncture points, although some will inevitably be stimulated because many of these begin and end on the feet.

Reflexology can also be done on the hands, but it is more common on the feet because it is easier, and less personal somehow. Some people prefer to have a little distance between themselves and the therapist.

The therapist will work on the whole foot, not just on isolated areas but if, for example you have a problem at menopause, they might spend more time on the area relating to the hormonal system.

❝ Reflexology can really fine-tune your hormones. If they're out of balance we can work on your feet to rebalance them. So it's particularly helpful for menopausal things like hot flushes. I've had a lot of success with that. You have to look at it holistically, so for example, with hot flushes, you would stimulate the points that relate to the female hormone system — the ovaries and uterus and so on — but at the same time you'd be working on the glands because they're all related in this big complicated hormonal structure. But you wouldn't leave anything out. You'd still work on the whole body, but just put extra emphasis on various areas. And you always do both feet.

A practising reflexologist ❞

The Association of Reflexologists:
www.aor.org.uk; info@aor.org.uk; tel 01823 351010

❝ I started seeing a reflexologist about four years ago because I was going through the menopause and getting fed up with having hot flushes and being so tired all the time. I always feel better when I have had a session with her, and my hot flushes are far less frequent since she started treating me. A while ago, she discovered that my thyroid needed some attention and she suggested I ask my doctor about this. The doctor did a test and it showed that my thyroid gland is basically wearing out, and that this needs to be checked regularly.

I take sea kelp tablets each day now which seem to do the trick, because last time it was checked it was OK. I don't think it would have been picked up at all otherwise, though, because I had no reason to see the doctor for anything else and I wouldn't have known myself. So now I feel I can prevent things getting any worse.

Janey, 55

"

ALEXANDER TECHNIQUE

The Alexander Technique is a sophisticated yet simple method of learning to use your body in the most effective way possible. Under a qualified practitioner, you learn to adjust and correct postural habits so that you can move with greater ease and efficiency. This helps to release unwanted tension, and so, among other things, it helps you to manage stress.

It was developed over a hundred years ago by a Tasmanian actor, Frederick Matthias Alexander, who found that his voice became hoarse during performances. As no medical causes could be found, he decided he must be doing something that caused him to strain his vocal organs. So he began to notice how he held his body when he spoke, and he noticed that his entire body posture affected his voice. He subsequently developed a technique to enable the whole body to be in balance and to move with ease.

66 People come to me with hot flushes and night sweats and they can't sleep. They find the work helps them. With Alexander work, it isn't that we tell you what to do. You learn through your own body what it wants to do, and how to release what interferes with your natural poise and balance.

If you are in pain we get to the root of why. We look at how the way you use your body causes you to have that pain. So rather than fixing it, we look at what it is that you are doing in your life that's causing your back, for example, to complain in that way. We teach you to listen to that, and make changes in the habits.

Alexander work is very much about being positive and not being pulled down. During the menopause your body is changing. There are physical, emotional and mental changes, and you can be pulled down by change. If you feel badly about yourself and what's happening to you, those negative thoughts will pull you down physically, emotionally and mentally. Making small physical adjustments enables you to start to think and feel more positive about the change. So having support at this time can be very valuable. Alexander work helps you to release upwards through the change.

So we help you to develop an awareness of your own body's balance and coordination, at a time when it might be disturbed. And therefore you come back into balance.

I like to think that at the menopause you are like a butterfly emerging from a chrysalis. It's a positive thing.

Valerie Willets, member of the Society of Teachers of the Alexander Technique

99

The Society of Teachers of Alexander Technique:
www.stat.org.uk; tel 0845 230 7878

Hypnotherapy

Hypnotherapy is a technique that uses something called hypnosis, which is an altered and heightened state of awareness. This is sometimes referred to as a trance state. You slip in and out of trance states throughout the day. For example, when you daydream and when you are at your most relaxed and comfortable. This is often when the best ideas pop into your mind.

Basically, there are two parts to the mind: the conscious, which is the thinking part, that deals with reason and logic, and the subconscious, which, among other things, houses all the information your conscious gives it to store, like memories and things it can't deal with immediately. (Many therapists use the term 'unconscious' instead of 'subconscious'.)

66 I think the menopause can exacerbate anxiety. For instance, a lot of us have children growing up with their own problems, and you have to cope with that. And then you have all your own stuff going on too. Someone suggested I see a hypnotherapist and it really helped.

Niki, 56

99

A hypnotherapist uses hypnosis to help you to relax your body and conscious mind so that your subconscious (or unconscious) can come forward easily, and your therapist can talk to it in order to bring about change.

Your therapist may:

- Introduce beneficial suggestions to the subconscious, which will help you to manage the changes you are experiencing, such as hot flushes

- Ask your subconscious questions to find out why you have a particular problem, such as anxiety or insomnia. Often, these issues may have been there all along, hidden deep in the subconscious, and the process of menopause has caused them to surface. So for example, if during menopause you start to get really anxious in certain situations where you didn't before, hypnotherapy can help you to get to the root of it, and fix it.

Hypnotherapy is very relaxing. It is very safe, and you cannot be made to do anything that you don't want to do.

General Hypnotherapy Standards Council:
www.GHSC.co.uk and www.general-hypnotherapy-register.com; tel 01590 683770

See: www.carolinecarrhypnotherapy.co.uk for hypnotherapy with me.

" I feel a lot more positive now. I was feeling so overwhelmed, and I was a bit of a mess really. I had four sessions and after each one I felt better, as if a weight had been lifted. And it's lasted. I feel much stronger now.
Billie, 53 **"**

Di

*Now 63, **Di**'s experience of the menopause led her to become qualified in various complementary therapies, and she has helped many women as a practitioner.*

"When I was 50 my periods stopped - just like that. I never had another one and I'd had no symptoms prior to that, except that every other period had been very slight. But then I started getting symptoms. The worst was the lack of sleep. I started to have hot flushes every half-an-hour during the day and night.

"At that stage I didn't know much about complementary therapies. But on a friend's recommendation I went to a Chinese acupuncturist and had a course of treatment, which was really good and it helped me out of that crisis time. The treatment was fairly intensive to start with. I went twice a week and he did electro acupuncture, where they put a little electrode into the needle and it's supposed to make it more powerful.

"Gradually over a few years the hot flushes died down altogether, and I don't get them any more now. But they went on for three or four years.

"Subsequently I've found out a lot more about complementary therapies, especially the use of herbs. Different ones work on different people, to different degrees, and at different stages. And you need to take them for a while to know whether you're getting any effect or not. A lot of people won't stick with things and I think companies make a fortune out of people buying a few weeks' supply and then just giving up. If I was going through all that again, my first port of call would be to go to a medical herbalist.

"Later on, I put on weight, which I'm still trying to lose. Somehow I just can't lose it. I did lots of exercise, ate less, drank less - still I put on the weight. And I noticed that my skin cleared up quite a lot.

"I never considered HRT at all because my mother had breast cancer, and I wasn't going to try anything that might increase my risk. But I can understand why people do. Had I been doing a job where I couldn't organise my time myself, I may have thought differently and taken the risk. As it is, I've always believed in looking after myself and keeping fit. I do Pilates and yoga, and that helps in all sorts of ways.

"To be honest, for me the menopause was just a drag. Nothing good came out of it really. Some women see it as a life-changing experience from which they benefit. I didn't at all. It was a complete nuisance. But I would advise any woman going through it to go to see a medical herbalist, and consider a therapy like acupuncture or reflexology in conjunction with that."

11

Food and nutrition

What you eat and drink has an impact on your health. Therefore it is likely to have an effect on how you feel before, during and after your menopause, and taking care early on may help to prevent some discomfort. For example, it's known that for some women, tea, coffee and alcohol can make hot flushes worse. And it makes sense to me that if you put rubbish into your body, you can expect to get rubbish service from it. Barbara Cox is a holistic nutritionist, whose story illustrates this.

  ❝I was Canadian champion skater for four years, and I ate absolute rubbish. I was sponsored by a large sweet company and so I lived mainly off their chocolate bars. By the age of 18 I was really unwell. I couldn't train and I suffered regularly with injury. It wasn't good. I basically went to bed for three days, because my body had just shut down. My mum was a pharmacist, and her friend was a nutritionist, so together they came up with a good plan of nutrition and removed all the junk food. And I got better.**❞**

Barbara Cox BSc (Hons), Dip Nat, CEO Nutrichef

Barbara now advises people on nutrition. She recognises how easy it is to reach for a salty or sweet unhealthy snack, especially when you are busy and on the go. But although this may be satisfying in the short term, it stores up problems for the future.

❝ Most sweet snacks like doughnuts and biscuits and chocolate bars have such a high sugar level that they do long-term damage. The sugar produces acid in the system, and when the body is acidic one of the defence mechanisms is to produce fat cells, which can be hard to work off. It also rots teeth, causes acne, puts extra stress on your liver, gives you constipation — the list is huge. These snacks are often full of hydrogenated fats and preservatives, and too much dairy produce too, which is not good.

Also, many people don't realise that there is a synergistic effect. For example, the combination of having a sweet chocolate bar and a Diet Coke together can cause all sorts of problems — it's a double whammy of sugar and artificial sweeteners, which, like sugar, bring their own set of health problems. There are alternatives that you can use which are much better for you, such as xylitol, which is a natural sugar from tree bark. It looks like white sugar, is granulated, very sweet, and is absolutely fine to use.

Too much salt is bad as well, and most people get all they need in their diet without needing to add any extra. The trouble is that salt and sugar are in so many things. Even some medications and high-street vitamins and mineral supplements contain them.

Barbara Cox BSc (Hons), Dip Nat, CEO Nutrichef **❞**

The following is a list of common junk foods and some better alternatives that Barbara recommends.

JUNK FOODS	BETTER CHOICES
Chocolate bars	Green & Black's chocolate – but only consume in moderation
Crisps	Vegetable crisps, spelt crackers, oat cakes, rice cakes, bread sticks
Chips	Home-made oven-baked wedges with the skin on
Cream cakes	Make your own cakes
Biscuits	Home-made oatmeal cookies and flapjacks
Sugar	Maple sugar, xylitol, Perfect Sweet*
Burgers	Home-made burgers with lean mince, soya mince, fresh tofu, mashed chickpeas or lentils, or home-made fish cakes.
Pizza	Home-made pizza. Make your own base and load it with fresh vegetables and non-dairy cheese
Cream	Soya cream
Sausages	Vegetarian sausages
*Perfect Sweet is a sugar alternative made from xylitol. If you have diabetes you can use this too. You can buy it at several large supermarket chains and health food shops. It is more expensive than sugar, but it is a health investment. See www.perfectsweet.co.uk	

I think it's easy to be put off making real changes to something as integral to your life as food, when it could involve using ingredients that you are not familiar with. Particularly if you lead a really busy life, and feel out of sorts because of menopausal changes too. Barbara recognises this and suggests that you should avoid making too many changes at once.

" You need to pace yourself to make changes to your diet. So when you remove one thing, replace it with something else. For example, replace salt with something like Himalayan sea salt which is much better and still contains 84 trace minerals. You can replace one thing one week, and another the next. So over a six-month period you will have done a complete lifestyle change and integrated it beautifully without any nutritional culture shock. It makes it easy, especially if you have children or grandchildren and everything else to take care of at the same time. It has to be done naturally and progressively. And you can re-route your regular supermarket shop – avoid going down the less healthy aisles you usually visit, and spend more time looking at home baking and 'free-from' items.

Barbara Cox BSc (Hons), Dip Nat, CEO Nutrichef "

Barbara also suggests that it is better to avoid too much dairy produce and to drink lots of water – at least 1.5 litres a day, because it helps to regulate the system. And she advocates using a range of cold-pressed oils, because these help to regulate hormones and lubricate joints. She especially recommends using flaxseed oil which has omega oils 3, 6 and 9 and is good for breast health, among other things.

Nibbling a variety of seeds, such as linseeds (the same as flaxseeds), hemp seeds or pumpkin seeds is great, because they contain lots of good oils. You might like to try mixing pumpkin, sunflower and sesame seeds, sprinkling them with soy sauce and roasting them in the oven.

If you are making changes to your diet and want to incorporate more seeds, I would recommend buying a good coffee grinder. That way, if you don't like the taste or texture of some of them, you can just grind them and add them to crumbles and cakes and things and you'd never know, yet still get the benefits. (I've never liked linseeds whole, and I detest the taste of the oil – but grinding them finely is a great way to deal with them.)

Barbara has created a recipe for HeaRTy muffins especially for readers of this book. Turn to page 211 to try them out yourself.

Avoid worrying and becoming obsessive about food. If you want to make changes, use Barbara's advice and do things in stages. And if you lapse, or find it tricky to stick to your decisions – so what? It doesn't matter. You can just carry on when you are ready. If you would like to see a nutritionist for help through the menopause, whether it is to relieve symptoms or for advice on your diet generally, the contacts below will be able to advise you.

The British Association of Nutritional Therapists (BANT):
www.bant.org.uk; tel 08706 061284

The Institute for Optimum Nutrition:
www.ion.ac.uk; tel 020 8614 7800

Barbara Cox:
BSc (Hons), Dip Nat, CEO Nutrichef:
www.nutrichef.co.uk; barbara@nutrichef.co.uk;
tel 0845 366 9900

SUPPLEMENTS

Supermarkets and health food shops are full of supplements – vitamins, minerals, herbs, extracts of various things, and so on. And there are specially created packs designed to help you through various stages of your life, such as when you are a baby, a toddler, a child, at puberty, and when you are premenstrual. There are packs to help you when you're pregnant, when you are giving birth to the baby, after you've had the baby, when you are breastfeeding it, and to help you to survive when it's growing up. And there are packs to help you as you approach the menopause, after you have had your menopause, and into old age.

Over the years I must have spent literally hours pondering over some of these products. I was able to get advice in some of the more specialist shops, depending on who was on duty at the time. Often, when I was approaching the menopause, I felt I 'needed something' just to give me some 'oomph'. So I usually came away with a multivitamin and mineral that was on special offer. I took them – but I was never really sure if they had helped. I wonder how many of you can identify with this? My guess is that it may be quite a few of you.

And the marketing on some of these is phenomenal. In one health magazine I came across there were adverts for products which claimed that: 'Thousands of women worldwide have discovered…', 'Scientists have proved that…', 'This wonderful product from [another country] has now come to the UK to help women…', 'Research has shown that the effective combination of [however many] minerals will boost your level of…' Most of these products contained something from plants or trees.

It's worth remembering that just because something is natural it doesn't necessarily mean that it's safe. So be careful where you buy products from.

The idea behind taking supplements at the menopause is that, having recognised that your body is missing certain things, you give it what it needs to support it through the transition naturally, bearing in mind that what you need will change as you progress through. The advice is to listen to your body and if you notice that something isn't right, then seek help.

> The first thing that I do with a person who comes to me for a consultation is a health analysis, and I talk to the client about their diet. The health analysis is a questionnaire which asks lots of health and lifestyle questions, and that pinpoints to me the particular areas in their health which are very low. We can work on those, using organic vitamins and minerals to boost those systems up. The body is only as strong as its weakest system. This takes about an hour. I keep in contact with clients and see them again in three months to reassess the situation.
>
> People tend to pick up all sorts of supplements in the shops based on what they see and hear in the media, and they don't really know what they're getting. This is why I can lead them to the right products, because the health analysis is very visual — people can see for themselves why I am recommending a particular supplement. Everyone has different needs, so we work to get the right combination for them. One size does not fit all as far as health is concerned.
>
> Dinah Smith, formerly a nurse, now a natural health adviser

Dinah stresses the importance of taking natural and organically sourced supplements which are tested sufficiently to make sure that they are of high enough quality and potency to be effective, and that they are pure, and not contaminated in any way, such as with radiation or dirt. Black cohosh is an example of this.

> **“**There's been a lot of media attention about black cohosh being dangerous for the liver. But it's not the black cohosh itself – it's the herb that grows with it that causes liver problems. Unfortunately, many companies don't test to see if this second herb is in the raw black cohosh that they receive from the growers. So it's important to make sure that the source is organic and natural, and that it's been tested to check that there are no traces of other herbs or contamination of any kind.
>
> Dinah Smith, natural health adviser **”**

It is also important to understand that health and fitness are two different things:

Health is when your immune system is high, your energy is great, and your vitality is good. Your body can throw off infections quickly.

Fitness means that you are just that – fit. You may have the ability to run a marathon, have fantastic stamina and endurance and good muscle strength, but that doesn't mean that you're healthy.

You can be healthy, but that doesn't mean to say that you are fit, and vice versa. It is important to achieve a balance between the two.

BLOOD SUGAR LEVELS

Keeping your blood sugar level in balance is important because it affects how you function. For example, it affects your energy levels, moods and weight. Therefore it has an impact on pre-menstrual tension and menopausal symptoms such as hot flushes.

Dinah Smith suggests that you start the day with protein to take your blood sugar levels to the optimum zone and keep them there all day. After that, eat small, regular meals to keep your blood sugar levels balanced. These should be low-glycaemic foods like brown rice, brown pasta, fruit, vegetables, and salads. Glycaemic means the speed at which, and the way that, your body breaks down simple sugars. Low glycaemic breaks them down slowly, high glycaemic breaks them down very quickly, and therefore raises your blood sugar level quickly.

You may crave sugar before a period. That's because your blood sugar level gets out of balance. So if you eat something sweet, you'll find that the refined sugar breaks down very quickly into simple sugars which release glucose into your bloodstream. Therefore you get a quick spurt of energy, and then your blood sugar level drops very quickly, which makes your body crave sugar again. Dinah also extols the benefits of liquorice.

❝ Not sugary liquorice sweets, but liquorice root. The herb liquorice is fantastic – put a couple of drops on your tongue and it takes away the craving for sweetness, and it regulates the blood sugar levels. Chomping on an old-fashioned liquorice root is quite good, but it 's easier to have it as a liquid or a capsule. Liquorice also lifts your blood pressure, so it 's a good, natural way of raising it if you need to.

Liquorice and keeping my sugar levels at the right level has been life-changing for me. I don't crave sweet processed foods at all, and my food choices are much healthier. And I 'm happier. My moods are better. I wake up in the morning feeling much brighter. All those things have an effect. My vitality is so much better than it ever was.

"

Dinah Smith, natural health adviser

Liquorice tips

If you have high blood pressure you shouldn't eat liquorice. It's worth taking a healthy snack with you when you are out, to avoid being 'too busy to eat'. That way you will keep your blood sugar level up and maintain a reasonable balance.

OESTROGENS AND PHYTOESTROGENS

There are different types of oestrogen:

- Oestrogen that you make in your body. You need this to survive.

- Oestrogen that you get from foods – proteins such as soya, for example, and plants. These are also called phytoestrogens and are quite weak.

- Oestrogen that is in things like plastics, and certain foods (processed foods, for example). These are bad for you because they can get into your hormone receptors and cause havoc.

Eating foodstuffs like soya, which contains good oestrogen, puts a barrier around your hormone receptors and prevents the bad oestrogen getting through. It may be that eating a diet high in phytoestrogens lessens the unpleasant effects of the menopause. So foods could include soya beans and tofu, pulses, linseed, citrus fruit and cereals.

> **❝** There are hormones in so many things now, even in plastic drinks bottles. These oestrogens aren't good for us but they help to keep the plastic supple. As the bottles become warm they release oestrogens into the drink. And cows are fed hormones which get into the milk we drink. A lot of the time we have an overload of oestrogens in our bodies, so we need to balance that because a lot of our hormone problems can be traced to oestrogen overload.
>
> But there are things that you can do naturally to put your body back in balance, especially with the help of experts who know how to do this. Also, be sensible, and do things in moderation. An excess of anything is bad for you. And it's important to take control of your own health.
>
> Dinah Smith, natural health adviser **❞**

Dinah Smith:
dinah@mad4organics.com; www.mad4organics.com;
tel 01202 474343

ALCOHOL

Current advice is that women should not regularly drink more than two to three units of alcohol a day. You may think you are drinking one or two units, but you could be drinking considerably more, depending on the strength of the drink (that's the percentage of alcohol in it), and the amount you have. So, for example, a *small* glass of 12.5% wine equates to 1.6 units of alcohol.

Many pubs serve wine in far bigger glasses, and if you pour a drink yourself you may pour generously.

All the road signs and adverts that say, 'Think! Don't drink and drive' mean exactly that. Although there is a *legal* limit for drinking before driving, this is not the *safe* limit.

The safe limit is not to drink any alcohol at all. And the reason for this is that alcohol starts to affect your judgement as soon as it gets into your system. It slows your reaction time. You may feel as if it has the opposite effect, but that is not so. And if your hormones are erratically rushing through your system anyway – well, there you have a potentially very dangerous cocktail.

Too much alcohol can affect your ability to retain and recall information. You may want to consider this if you find that forgetfulness is one of the changes that exasperates you as you go through the menopause.

One unit of alcohol takes about an hour to 'leave' the body, although you don't count the first hour after the first drink. But that is an average guide. Everyone is different, and many people may need considerably more time to become 'alcohol-free' (although there is usually a tiny amount of alcohol present in the body anyway, for example from fruit as it ferments). Illness and medications can affect this too. And, of course, so can hormones.

Time is the only thing that sobers you up. Your liver needs time to break down the alcohol. Strong black coffee won't do it.

Be informed about alcohol. It might be tempting to reach for a glass or two of something when you're feeling tired/down/ want to unwind/need a bit of confidence, and that's fine, but it is now known that the cumulative effect of drinking lots of alcohol isn't good for you.

The Drinkaware Trust:
This is a great organisation that can give you masses more information on alcohol, units and its effects on health generally: www.drinkaware.co.uk; tel 020 7907 3700

Dinah

Dinah Smith, *natural health adviser, has contributed to this book in the food and nutrition section. This is her story.*

"A few years ago I went to the doctor because I had a problem with the discs in my back. I was given steroid injections and the last one I had put my body into shock and caused my pituitary gland to shut down. This meant that I went through the menopause from that moment. So, from having perfectly normal, regular periods, with no problems whatsoever - within six months I'd gone through the menopause. I was 42 at the time.

"I had no idea I'd gone through the menopause. I knew I wasn't well, but didn't know why. I was trying for another baby at the time and was having regular visits to the fertility clinic. I only knew I'd gone through the menopause because the doctor told me. That came as a great shock and, understandably, was a great disappointment. He said there was no way I could get pregnant under my own steam now. I'd have to use egg donation.

"Then I was put onto HRT because I was so young, to protect my bones and so on. I had four different types of HRT and each one made me nauseous and generally unwell. Then a friend introduced me to natural remedies, and I was able to use a natural alternative to HRT - a combination of herbs, vitamins and minerals – that helped my body ease through the menopause on its own.

"Within two months I completely changed my health around. It probably took three or four months to get the full benefits. It was fantastic. It changed my husband's life as well, because my going through the menopause so very quickly affected him too.

"The result was that I started losing weight, my energy levels went up, and all the symptoms went away. The hot flushes and the anxiety went, I was sleeping better, my skin improved and I felt so much healthier. Friends and family saw what I was doing and started to ask questions about it. So I started researching natural products a lot more, and started talking to groups of women who were going through menopause, to help them to make their own informed choices as to how to 'manage' the menopause.

"Now I'm fine, very healthy. My skin has never been so good, or my hair – everything is better than it has been for years. I'm not saying medication isn't right – I believe that there's always a place for medication, but if your body is healthy, then you are less likely to need medical intervention."

part four

Supporting others

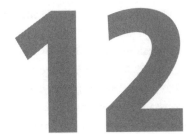

Unity is strength

HELPING YOUR PARTNER GO THROUGH THE MENOPAUSE

Menopause can be a really tricky time for partners, and you may experience all sorts of emotions yourself. This isn't just 'a woman's thing'. You will be going through your partner's menopause with her. So it's helpful to find out about it and become as informed as you can, so that you have some understanding about what you might expect.

You may find that your partner behaves differently, and does some things that, to you, seem ridiculous. Sometimes she may react in unusual ways. Perhaps she seems ultra-sensitive about things, and maybe she cries a lot. Maybe, for the first time ever, she seems depressed. She may go off you completely for a while.

She might be irritated and snappy and you don't know why. She may lose interest in sex completely. Perhaps she feels guilty and vulnerable. Maybe she says horrible things to you, and then wants a cuddle – then she pushes you away. Perhaps she's concerned that she's ill and is frightened, but won't talk about it. Maybe her constant apologising drives you mad. You might be at your wits' end and have no idea what to do for the best, how you can help, or who you could talk to about it.

Many men are uncomfortable talking about their feelings. Some men find it tricky to identify the feelings they experience, so they bottle them up. But that's not good. You need to be able to express how you feel, somehow. It might be that you and your partner share similar emotions, but this could be for different reasons. For example:

YOU BOTH MIGHT FEEL	YOU FEEL THIS WAY BECAUSE	SHE FEELS THIS WAY BECAUSE
Confused and bewildered	You don't know why she is reacting and behaving as she does. Sometimes she seems fine, and sometimes she doesn't.	She has to come to terms with her menopause, and all the physical changes that entails, and all the emotions that triggers.
Worried, insecure, vulnerable	You fear she is rejecting you. You are worried about her and you don't know what to do.	She fears you will 'go off her' and ultimately reject her, especially if she feels unattractive, moody and irritable, gets hot flushes and night sweats, can't sleep, doesn't want sex – or if she does, takes ages to reach orgasm (if at all).

Uncertain	You don't know how long this will last, and if this might mean permanent changes in your relationship.	She's not sure what to expect next and she has no idea how long the menopause process might last for her. And she is uncertain as to how this might affect your relationship.
Lonely and alone	You don't know what to do for the best, who to talk to, or how to help her.	She might feel lonely and alone because she feels misunderstood. She might desperately want to talk to you about how she feels, but may fear your reaction.
Incompatible	You want sex, and she doesn't. Or perhaps you don't want sex and she wants it more than ever.	She doesn't want sex, and you do. Or perhaps she wants sex more than ever, and you want it less than you used to.
Rejected and unloved	You feel she doesn't care about you any more. She doesn't show you affection, and she doesn't want sex, so you are at a loss as to what to do.	She wants to be shown affection. She craves intimacy. She wants spontaneous non-sexual cuddles and caresses, but you aren't supplying them. She wants reassurance that she is loved and understood.
Miserable	You don't know how long you can take this. Things have changed.	She sometimes feels lousy physically, and she's fed up with it. And she feels emotionally wobbly and she's had enough of that too.

So talk to her – and listen to her. Support her in the best way that you can. Avoid saying things like, 'I don't know what's the matter with you' or 'My mother/sister was never like this, so I don't know why you are.' That won't help.

Your partner is her own unique self, which is probably why you are with her anyway, and she will experience her menopause in her own way.

66 Most of my friends are at various stages of the menopause. They're all strong, successful women, but suddenly they are being sort of wimpish about things. It's the emotions running riot. Things that normally you'd brush off are a big issue. It must be tough for their husbands too. It's made me think, because I notice that several of my mother's friends got divorced after about 25 years of marriage. And there were others where the marriage survived, but their husbands had affairs. It makes you wonder if that coincides with the menopause. There may have been all sorts of reasons – it could be that the children were of an age that the mother felt that she could go. Or maybe a loss of sex drive, feeling inadequate, arguments possibly because of the emotional ups and downs. It would be interesting to see statistics of all the affairs, divorces and separations around the time of the menopause.
Rebecca, 43 99

One thing that's unlikely to help is if you decide you've had enough and you leave. And it is unlikely to help either of you if you close yourself down and shut yourself off from her. But be mindful of the fact that you may have your own issues around this time. Your life could be changing too, outside of your relationship. You might have your own external pressures, and you may have your own emotional issues anyway. Perhaps your partner has always been there for you, but now seems more vulnerable, or is unable to give you the attention that you need.

Tell each other how you feel. Make the best attempt to understand each other. If you are not quite sure how best to broach the subject, you could try using a loose format which avoids being harsh or blundering, or disrespectful, and enables you both to be clear:

1. Say what the situation is.

2. Say how you feel about it.

3. Say what you want to happen and how this will benefit you both.

So, for example, it might go something like this:

1. 'I notice that you seem to be upset a lot at the moment . . .'

2. '... and I feel helpless, because I don't know what's bothering you.'

3. 'It'd be great to talk about how you feel so that I can try and understand. Then maybe I can help you to feel better.'

This makes it clear and leaves it open enough for a conversation to start. It also shows that you are noticing and taking an interest.

When starting a conversation that could potentially be quite delicate, it's best to start with a question that is likely to get more than 'yes' or 'no' for an answer.

You might say something like the following – the words in italics are good ones to use to help someone to open up:

Q: *Tell me about* your day
A: It was awful. (Or you might get lots more information at this point.)

Q: *How* was it awful?
A: I don't want to talk about it. (Again, you may get lots more information at this point.)

Q: OK, well I'm here if you do. (And then be inquisitive.) *I'm just wondering* what's going on for you, because you don't seem your normal self . . .
A: Well, this happened and that happened and I felt . . .

On the other hand you might get a response like this:
A: Look, I don't want to talk about it. Now shut up and leave me alone.

These approaches may or may not work for you, but at least they'll give you a chance, and you'll have tried. And keep trying. One day's response might be totally different from that of the next day. And another thing to bear in mind – avoid using the word 'you' too much, or that will sound as if you are apportioning blame.

If you find conversations with your partner really tricky at the moment, you could ask for help. Avoid letting pride get in the way – ask appropriate people for advice. Some people have found that couple counselling has been really useful for them. After all, that's what it's there for – to help.

LOOKING AFTER YOURSELF DURING YOUR PARTNER'S MENOPAUSE

While doing your best to understand and support your partner, you need to look after yourself too. So be gentle with yourself. Allow yourself to talk about how you feel, because this is so important for your own health.

If you've become informed about the menopause, you will have a good understanding of how tricky and how lengthy a time this can be for both of you.

You may want to share your thoughts and feelings with someone other than your partner, and discuss your concerns privately with someone outside of your relationship. Many people are flattered if you confide in them, and are glad to be of help, but of course you need to pick that person wisely, and be sure it's someone you can trust. So it could be a good friend, a family member or a work colleague.

If the thought of 'opening up' to anyone you know makes you cringe, then there are plenty of professionals to turn to, and it may be more appropriate for you to do so. And you can always ask your doctor for advice – especially if you have particular concerns. Sharing your thoughts, feelings and concerns with another person can bring a huge sense of relief.

Keep upbeat and positive. Avoid being dragged down by your partner's menopause. So if she is feeling low, listen to her, support her and help her, but understand that you do not need to feel low too. Similarly if she is crotchety and mean, avoid being hurt. Practise letting her unkind words bounce off you (unless she has good reason to say them). She probably feels guilty, and hates herself for giving you so much grief.

Many women feel that they just cannot control some of these outbursts as their hormones rush riotously through their body. Well, you may not be able to change the way your partner thinks, feels or behaves, but you can choose how this affects you.

Always be prepared to listen, and to express compassion and love and respect. But hang on to your sense of self, and keep a sense of perspective. The menopause doesn't last for ever, so enjoy the best times now, and look forward to the future. There'll probably be many times when you'll both look back and laugh.

Above all, be gentle with each other. Love each other and support one another, and talk together. Tell each other how you feel. And move into the next phase of your lives positively and with enthusiasm.

Appendices

A brief survival guide

ATTITUDE

Remember, your best self-help tool is your positive attitude. Keep upbeat and optimistic, because this will help you every step of the way. But be realistic too. If you need help, do ask for it.

And bear this word in mind:
WAFER. This stands for Water, Avoid, Food, Exercise, Relax – all great tips to help you survive the menopause, whichever stage you are at.

Water
Drink lots of it.

Avoid
Smoking, too much caffeine and alcohol.

Food
Eat a well-balanced diet of good, nutritious food with less junk food.

Exercise
Enjoy your exercise, whatever you choose to do. You may like to do an activity like yoga or tai chi, or you may enjoy the gym. But there's no need to overdo it – just some brisk, aerobic walking

a few times a week will suffice. If you're not used to exercising, build it up slowly until it becomes an enjoyable habit rather than a chore.

Relax

Make an effort to relax. This means relaxing your body properly each day, which will help your mind to relax too. Relaxing your mind and body properly can only ever do you good, even if you are not aware of the immediate benefits. A really effective way to do this is to find somewhere comfortable, then sit or lie down, and progressively tense and release the muscles in your body. You can work from the tips of your toes all the way up to the top of your head, tensing and relaxing each bit in turn, for example, toes, feet, calves, thighs, and so on.

Doing a progressive relaxation like this can take practice, and if you're not used to doing it you may find that you wriggle and twitch at first. But regular practice of this is well worth the effort. Among other benefits, it enables you to identify where in your body you carry stress. And once you are aware, you can release it. It's often much easier to do a progressive relaxation if you can listen to someone talking you through it, because this encourages you to focus.

Visit my website – www.carolinecarr.com – to download a relaxation routine.

And give yourself a mental break sometimes. Let your mind drift into a place that pleases you. It could be to a beach with smooth white sand, or to a beautiful garden with trees and flowers, or maybe to a wood with a stream or a waterfall. Or perhaps to a fabulous room, or a temple. Choose wherever you wish. Spend a few minutes 'being there'. Enjoy the experience and notice colours, sounds, scents and tastes. Take pleasure from this wonderful daydream, and return there whenever you want some time for yourself. Use it like a comfort blanket. It's yours. No-one else can intrude there, unless you allow them to.

There's a saying: *a change is as good as a rest.* By doing this exercise, you give your mind a pleasant change, and that in itself is a mental rest.

Mental and physical relaxation helps to bring you back into balance – and that's the most important thing.

Helpful recipes

Triumphant Tofu Truffles

Many of us adore chocolate, and probably crave it from time to time. I certainly do, and I particularly like rich and delicious truffles. However, I don't like the thought of what's in them as they usually contain a fair percentage of fatty stuff like cream and butter, which I prefer to avoid.

So I have invented a truffle which contains tofu (soya bean curd), and no fat other than that already present in the chocolate that is used. I am amazed at the success of this. OK, there are probably other recipes, but I've not found one yet. So I am triumphant. Finally, here's a chocolate truffle that may actually be quite good for you. Try the recipe and see what you think:

Ingredients (for about 24 truffles):
  1 block of firm tofu (about 200-250g)
  1 100gm bar of plain chocolate – Green & Black's 70% is good
  1 dessertspoon of plain cocoa
  1 teaspoon/dessertspoon of honey (or you could use Perfect Sweet)
  1 teaspoon of molasses
  Extras might be:
  1 tablespoon of ground almonds, or
  1 tablespoon of any chopped nuts, or
  a dash of whisky, brandy, rum or liqueur or essence

● Melt the chocolate.

● Whiz the tofu in a food processor with the cocoa.

- Add the honey and molasses, and any extras you might fancy.

- Add the melted chocolate.

- Mould into truffle-sized balls and roll them in cocoa.

You could dip the truffles in melted chocolate instead of rolling in cocoa if you wish. They freeze well too.

It's worth experimenting with these until you get them just right for you. After all, a little of what you fancy does you good!

HeaRTy Muffins

Barbara Cox, CEO of Nutrichef, created these HeaRTy muffins especially for readers of this book. You might like to try them. They're delicious – but they are nothing like a light fluffy cream cake, so be prepared for something quite different. It doesn't matter if you don't have *all* the seeds – I've made them without hemp seeds or ginger and they are still good.

Ingredients

> 100 gm rice flour
> 50 gm each of sunflower seeds, pumpkin seeds, linseeds, hemp seeds, sesame seeds, flaked almonds, pine nuts, Perfect Sweet
> 1 teaspoon baking powder
> 100 gm each dried cranberries and dried apricots
> 1 inch fresh stem ginger, grated
> ½ teaspoon each nutmeg and cinnamon
> 1 tablespoon molasses
> 3 tablespoonapple juice
> 400ml-450ml unsweetened soya milk

- Pre-heat oven to 190C.

- Grind 25gm each of sunflower seeds, pumpkin seeds and linseeds.

- Mix all dry ingredients in a bowl.

- Add apple juice and soya milk and stir until the mixture is of a thick, dropping consistency.

- Arrange muffin/fairy cake liners on tray and fill with 1 tbsp of mixture.

- Bake for 15–25 minutes, or until done.

Note: muffins are meant to be of dense consistency and are better served warm.

Useful contacts

CONTACTS FOR MENOPAUSE INFORMATION

The British Menopause Society
www.thebms.org.uk
admin@thebms.org.uk
tel 01628 890199

The Daisy Network
For those who experience premature menopause
www.daisynetwork.org.uk
daisy@daisynetwork.org.uk

Menopause Matters
www.menopausematters.co.uk
info@menopausematters.co.uk

NHS Direct www.nhsdirect.nhs.uk
24-hour helpline 0845 46 47

Women's Health Concern (WHC)
www.womens-health-concern.org
tel 01628 478 473
confidential advice line 0845 123 2319

CONTACTS FOR SPECIFIC ISSUES AND TREATMENTS

Mental health

Alzheimer's Society
www.alzheimers.org.uk
tel 020 7423 3500

Anxiety UK
For all sorts of help with anxiety, panic and phobias
www.anxietyuk.org.uk
info@anxietyuk.org.uk
tel 08444 775 774
or 0161 227 9898

The Depression Alliance
For those affected by depression
www.depressionalliance.org
tel 0845 123 23 20

Samaritans www.samaritans.org
24-hour helpline 08457 90 90 90

MIND
Provides a range of information and leaflets on all aspects of mental health
www.mind.org
0845 766 1063

Sane
www.sane.org.uk
020 7375 1002

British Association for Counselling and Psychotherapy (BACP)
www.bacp.ck.uk
0870 443 5252

United Kingdom Council for Psychotherapy (UKCP)
www.psychotherapy.org.uk
020 7014 9955

Complementary Therapy associations

Alliance of Registered Homeopaths
www.a-r-h.org
tel 08700 736339

Society of Homeopaths
www.homeopathy-soh.org
tel 0845 450 6611

Aromatherapy Council
www.aromatherapycouncil.co.uk
tel 0870 774 3477

Association of Reflexologists
www.aor.org.uk
info@aor.org.uk
tel 01823 351010

The Association of Traditional Chinese Medicine (UK) (ATCM)
www.atcm.co.uk
info@atcm.co.uk
tel 020 8951 3030

Ayurvedic Practitioners' Association
www.apa.uk.com
tel 07985 984146

British Acupuncture Council
www.acupuncture.org.uk
info@acupuncture.org.uk
tel 020 8735 0400

British Association of Nutritional Therapists (BANT)
www.bant.org.uk
tel 08706 061284

Institute for Optimum Nutrition
www.ion.ac.uk
tel 020 8614 7800

National Candida Society
www.candida-society.org

The National Institute of Medical Herbalists (NIMH)
www.nimh.org.uk
info@nimh.org.uk
tel 01392 426022

National Osteoporosis Society
www.nos.org.uk
tel 0845 450 0230

British Heart Foundation.
www.bhf.org.uk
Heart helpline 0300 330 3311

Society of Teachers of Alexander Technique:
www.stat.org.uk
tel 0845 230 7878

General Hypnotherapy Register
www.general-hypnotherapy-register.com
tel 01590 683770

General Hypnotherapy Standards Council
www.GHSC.co.uk

Voice Care Network UK,
For advice about voice care and workshops
www.voicecare.org.uk
info@voicecare.org.uk
tel 01926 864000

Complementary health practitioners mentioned in this book

Barbara Cox
CEO Nutrichef
www.nutrichef.co.uk
barbara@nutrichef.co.uk
tel 0845 366 9900

Caroline Carr Hypnotherapy
www.carolinecarrhypnotherapy.co.uk
caroline@carolinecarrhypnotherapy.co.uk
tel 01202 731385

Claire Short, nutritional adviser,
cshort124@googlemail.com
tel 07982 254362

Dinah Smith, natural health adviser
www.mad4organics.com
dinah@mad4organics.com
tel 01202 474343

Other

The Drinkaware Trust
For all alcohol-related matters
www.drinkaware.co.uk
tel 020 7907 3700

Dry eyes
www.clarymist.co.uk
tel 08450 60 60 70

Chillow pad
www.chillow.co.uk
info@soothsoft.co.uk
tel 08700 117174

Hula hoop
www.valentinesports.co.uk
02392 428825

INDEX